# Empowering Birth

## The Role of Midwifery and Physician Collaboration in Modern Maternity Care.




By Dr. Michael J. Hervey II MD

**With Contributions From:**

Ellie Tan MSN, CNM, WHNP-BC

Melissa Sue Christenson MSN, CNM, WHNP-BC

Kim Flanders DNP, CNM, FACNM

Michelle M. Davis DNP, NNP, CNM

Makenzie C. Bailey MSN, CNM, WHNP-BC

Tracy L. Burns MSN, CNM

**Edits provided by:**

Monte G. Merrell MD

Krunal Patel MD, MFM

ISBN eBook: 979-8-8693-4816-6
ISBN Softcover: 979-8-8693-4812-8
ISBN Hardcover: 979-8-8693-4978-1

Printed in the United States Published by USA Publishing Hub

# Dedication

To the midwives, physicians, and all who dedicate their lives to the work of birth— thank you for standing at the front lines of life itself, for bringing skill, strength, and heart to moments that demand all three.

To the mothers— who risk everything, who give everything, who cross the threshold between life and death to bring new life into the world— your sacrifice is seen, honored, and never forgotten.

This book is for you. For the hard nights, the quiet victories, the losses that broke you, and the triumphs that remade you.

May we never take for granted the cost of life. May we honor birth with the respect, care, and unity it deserves. And may we always remember: It is through your courage that the future is born.

# Introduction

She was a firecracker — a petite redhead, sharp as a whip, 32 years young, standing at the edge of motherhood. Her husband, equally composed yet brimming with silent strength, never left her side. Together, they were a force — a true power couple.

Their pregnancy journey had been smooth, almost deceptively so, with only one dark cloud: thrombocytopenia — low platelets. She wanted, more than anything, a natural birth. And because her numbers weren't dangerously low, we didn't interfere. Still, we all knew the unspoken rule: if the platelets fell too far, an epidural wouldn't be an option. At her 36-week check-up, her counts hovered between 101 and 110. Good enough. Safe — for now.

Then came the moment. She arrived at the hospital, 40 weeks and six days pregnant, contracting and fierce. Her water broke almost the moment she walked through the door. The starting gun fired, and there was no turning back.

Reserved, determined, unwavering — she placed her faith in herself, in her husband, in us.

As the rituals of care began, we ran her labs. And when the results came back, the air in the room shifted: platelets at 70,000. Too low for an epidural. Too late for anything but raw strength.

She clenched her fists, took a deep breath, and said the words that sealed her fate: *Let's do this.* No medication. No shortcuts. Just willpower, love, and the long road ahead.

She labored for two days. Forty-eight hours of relentless contractions, of summoning strength from places no one could see. When she began to falter, I checked her. Complete. It was time. The final gauntlet: pushing.

We pushed together — her husband, myself, and this fierce woman who refused to give up. For nearly two hours, she battled against exhaustion, against the limits of her body. Her fiery spirit, the one that had carried her so far, flickered and began to dim.

Tears streamed down her face. She gasped that she had nothing left. Two days. No sleep. No relief. And the finish line still out of reach.

Her husband — hair matted, t-shirt soaked in sweat — looked at me with pleading eyes. I reached into the empty bag of tricks I carried, heart pounding. There was only one thing left to do.

I hit the SOS. The midwives answered. Like warriors entering a battlefield, they crossed the threshold, and I gave the call: *Healthy pregnancy. Low platelets. No epidural. Two days of labor. Two hours of pushing. She's got heart — but she needs help.*

Without hesitation, they moved. Flying cowgirls. Hip squeezes. Side-lying releases. Rebozo lifts. Coaching. Commanding. Championing. The room shifted — it became electric, alive, pulsing with the collective will of women who refused to let one of their own fall.

Something *sacred* happened in that room — a bond, a battle cry without words. They would get her across the finish line. She would not fall. Not here. Not now.

And then — an hour later — through tears, sweat, and something greater than any of us could name, she delivered her baby. A beautiful, full-term, healthy baby. Minimal tearing. Minimal blood loss. Maximum triumph.

The room erupted — not in noise, but in soul. Exhilaration. Awe. Gratitude.

# Contents

# Chapter 1
# Midwifery in Healthcare and The Historical Evolution of Midwifery

Midwifery has a deep-rooted history that dates back to ancient civilizations, where women were primarily responsible for providing care during childbirth. In ancient Egypt, Greece, and Rome, midwives played essential roles, attending births and assisting with postpartum care. Midwifery was often passed down from generation to generation, with knowledge gained through observation and practical experience rather than formal education. As societies evolved, so did the practice of midwifery, but its fundamental goal—supporting women during childbirth—remained consistent.

In the Middle Ages and the Renaissance, midwifery continued as a female-led profession, although it often faced challenges from emerging medical practices. The rise of obstetrics in the 18th and 19th centuries, particularly with the development of medicalized childbirth, began to shift childbirth from the home to hospitals, pushing midwifery into the background in many parts of the Western world. However, midwives remained integral to childbirth in many rural and underserved communities where doctors were scarce. This trend led to a polarization in maternal care, with physicians often managing high-risk cases and midwives handling normal, uncomplicated births.

In the 20th century, midwifery was revived in several countries as part of a broader movement to humanize childbirth. Influenced by feminist ideals and increasing interest in natural birth options, midwives regained prominence, particularly in places like the U.K., New Zealand, and parts of the U.S. Established professional bodies like the American College of Nurse-Midwives (ACNM) in 1955 helped formalize the profession, leading to greater recognition of midwives as key players in maternity care. This historical journey underscores the enduring importance of midwifery, highlighting its adaptability and resilience.

## The Evolution of Midwifery

Midwifery has evolved significantly over centuries, transitioning from a tradition-based practice rooted in community care to a highly specialized and regulated profession. Historically, midwives were integral to childbirth in nearly every culture, relying on experience, intuition, and shared knowledge passed down through generations. With the advent of medicalized childbirth in the 19th and 20th centuries, midwifery faced stigmatization and a decline in many regions as obstetrics gained prominence. However, the midwifery model of care has experienced a resurgence in recent decades, driven by a growing recognition of its holistic, patient-centered approach and its proven role in improving maternal and neonatal outcomes. Midwives are acknowledged as essential contributors to maternity care, offering a blend of time-honored practices and evidence-based medical expertise.

## Types of Midwives and Their Roles

Midwifery encompasses several distinct types of practitioners, each with unique scopes of practice, settings, and training pathways.

1. **Certified Nurse-Midwives (CNMs) are advanced-practice registered nurses who primarily provide care** in hospitals and clinics, often collaborating with obstetricians. They are licensed healthcare providers who manage pregnancies, births, and postpartum care and are authorized to prescribe medications in all 50 U.S. states.
2. **Certified Midwives (CMs):** They are similarly trained but do not hold a nursing degree; they focus on normal, low-risk pregnancies and often practice in birth centers or homes.
3. **Certified Professional Midwives (CPMs)** specialize in out-of-hospital births, with training emphasizing home and birth center settings.
4. **Traditional or Lay Midwives** operate outside formal medical systems, relying on apprenticeship-based or community-focused education.

## Training and Certification

The educational pathways for midwifery are uniquely diverse, reflecting the profession's broad spectrum of practice. CNMs, for example, must complete a nursing degree followed by a graduate-level midwifery program accredited by the Accreditation Commission for Midwifery Education (ACME). This rigorous training includes comprehensive obstetrics, gynecology, pharmacology, primary care, and clinical rotations coursework. CMs undergo similar training but without a nursing component. CPMs pursue a competency-based educational model, which includes clinical experience and certification through the North American Registry of Midwives (NARM). Each pathway emphasizes integrating evidence-based care, focusing on physiologic childbirth, patient autonomy, and collaborative practice.

## Regulation and Collaboration with Medical Boards

Regulations from various professional and medical organizations shape midwives' roles and responsibilities. CNMs and CMs are nationally certified and recognized by entities like the American College of Nurse-Midwives (ACNM) and often work under the guidelines of nursing boards or state medical boards. They collaborate closely with organizations such as the American College of Obstetricians and Gynecologists (ACOG) to ensure their practices align with current medical standards. Prescription authority is a defining feature of CNMs and CMs, requiring additional pharmacology training and adherence to state and federal regulations. For CPMs and non-nurse midwives, recognition and integration into formal medical systems vary widely by state, with ongoing efforts to standardize their role and ensure access to their services.

## The Role of Midwives in Maternal Health

Each type of midwife plays a vital role in maternal health, addressing the diverse needs of expectant parents across various care settings. The choice of midwife often depends on individual health circumstances, preferences for childbirth environments, and the desired balance between natural approaches and medical interventions. Recognizing these distinctions helps expectant parents make informed decisions about their care. While this discussion primarily focuses on Certified Nurse Midwives (CNMs), it also considers other types of midwives within the community to foster understanding and collaboration.

## Midwives and OB-GYNs: Complementary Roles in Maternity Care Training

Midwives typically undergo specialized training in midwifery, focusing on prenatal care, childbirth, and postpartum support. CNMs often hold advanced nursing degrees, blending nursing and midwifery expertise. OB-GYNs, in contrast, are medical doctors who complete medical school and a residency in obstetrics and gynecology, equipping them to address complex medical and surgical needs in maternity care.

## Approach

Midwives emphasize a holistic and natural approach to childbirth, prioritizing minimal intervention and individualized care. OB-GYNs, while also capable of supporting natural births, are more inclined to incorporate medical interventions, when necessary, particularly in high-risk or emergencies. This complementary dynamic ensures families can access care tailored to their unique needs and preferences.

## Scope of Practice

Midwives typically manage low-risk pregnancies and births, ensuring safe, personalized care in both home and hospital settings. OB-GYNs are trained to handle high-risk pregnancies, complications, and surgical interventions such as cesarean deliveries. This distinction fosters a collaborative relationship, allowing patients to transition seamlessly between providers if complications arise.

## Desired Outcomes of Pregnancy

Achieving positive outcomes in pregnancy and childbirth requires a collaborative approach among providers, with a shared focus on the well-being of the mother and baby. Key outcomes include:

1. **Healthy Mother:** Ensuring the physical and mental health of the mother throughout pregnancy, delivery, and postpartum recovery.
2. **Healthy Baby:** Supporting the delivery of a healthy newborn, free from congenital abnormalities or significant complications.
3. **Successful Delivery:** Promoting a safe and uncomplicated delivery, whether vaginal or cesarean, with minimal intervention whenever possible.
4. **Positive Birth Experience:** Creating a satisfactory and empowering experience for the mother, aligning with her preferences, cultural values, and emotional needs.

5. **Postpartum Recovery:** Facilitating effective recovery for the mother, addressing both physical healing and emotional well-being.

6. **Breastfeeding Success:** Offering comprehensive support for initiating and maintaining breastfeeding if the mother breastfeeds.

7. **Bonding:** Encouraging strong emotional bonds between the mother, baby, and partner, fostering family cohesion.

8. **Supportive Environment:** Ensuring access to ongoing support from healthcare providers, family, and community resources to sustain the mother's and baby's well-being.

These outcomes highlight the importance of collaboration and mutual respect between midwives and OB-GYNs, reinforcing a healthcare system prioritizing safety, autonomy, and compassionate care for families.

The evolution and diversity of midwifery demonstrate its adaptability and enduring relevance in modern healthcare. By bridging the gap between traditional practices and contemporary medicine, midwives provide a model of care that prioritizes safety, respect, and the well-being of birthing individuals and their families.

# Chapter 2

# Current Role of Midwives in Hospital and Out-of-Hospital Settings

Midwives play a critical role in modern healthcare, providing comprehensive care for women throughout pregnancy, labor, birth, and postpartum. In both hospital and out-of-hospital settings, midwives serve as essential providers who advocate for women's health, focusing on personalized, low-intervention care when appropriate. Within hospital settings, Certified Nurse Midwives (CNMs) are increasingly integrated into maternity care teams, often working alongside obstetricians to provide holistic and collaborative care.

CNMs manage normal, low-risk pregnancies and births, usually prioritizing the natural birthing process. They promote techniques that minimize unnecessary interventions, such as labor induction or cesarean sections, while supporting women's preferences.

In many cases, CNMs are the primary care providers for pregnant women, with obstetricians stepping in only when medical complications arise. This approach ensures that women receive individualized attention, focusing on safety and evidence-based practices.

## The Shift Toward Out-of-Hospital Births

The growing demand for Certified Nurse-Midwives (CNMs) in the home birth and birth center settings reflects a significant cultural and professional shift in maternity care. Increasingly, individuals with high levels of education and medical literacy, as well as even healthcare professionals, are seeking personalized, patient-centered care outside the traditional hospital environment. This shift is fueled by a desire to avoid the routine medicalization of childbirth, including unnecessary interventions, while still ensuring safety and access to skilled care providers. CNMs, with their advanced training, ability to prescribe medications, and collaborative capabilities with obstetricians and hospitals, are uniquely positioned to meet this demand. Their presence in home and birth center settings offers a balance between evidence-based practice and the supportive, non-interventionist philosophy that these clients often prioritize.

Statistics further underscore this trend. According to the National Center for Health Statistics (NCHS), out-of-hospital births in the U.S. have been steadily increasing, rising from 1.26% in 2011 to 1.61% in 2021. This trend is even more pronounced among specific demographics, particularly highly educated individuals who are more likely to research and advocate for their birth preferences. Studies show that planned home births and birth center births with skilled providers, such as CNMs, result in lower rates of cesarean sections, fewer interventions, and higher maternal satisfaction compared to hospital births. For example, the National Birth Center Study II found that only 6% of low-risk women who planned to give birth in a birth center with midwife care required a cesarean delivery, compared to the national average of nearly 32%.

## Safety Considerations in Different Birth Settings

For low-risk pregnancies, planned home births, birth center births, and hospital births under midwifery care can have comparable fetal outcomes, though results vary by study. Research suggests that birth center births have perinatal mortality rates similar to low-risk hospital births. In contrast, home births may carry a slightly higher neonatal risk, particularly for first-time mothers. However, some large-scale studies report no significant difference in perinatal mortality between planned home and hospital births when attended by qualified providers. The safety of out-of-hospital births depends on risk assessment, provider experience, and emergency preparedness, including a clear plan for hospital transfer if needed. Consulting healthcare professionals is essential in choosing the safest birth setting.

This growing preference for out-of-hospital births aligns with broader healthcare trends emphasizing autonomy, shared decision-making, and individualized care. CNMs bring clinical expertise and credibility that reassures clients while bridging the gap between home birth or birth center care and hospital-based services. Their ability to handle complications, collaborate with physicians, and transition care seamlessly to hospitals when necessary enhances safety and trust in these settings.

## The Expanding Role of CNMs in Maternity Care

As this shift continues, the role of CNMs in out-of-hospital births is likely to expand further, driven by increasing awareness of the benefits of midwifery-led care and a growing demand for alternatives to conventional hospital births. Meeting this demand will require continued advocacy, policy changes to support midwifery practice in all settings, and investment in training programs to prepare CNMs for the unique challenges and opportunities of home and birth center care. This evolution not only reflects changing consumer preferences but also represents an opportunity to improve maternal and neonatal outcomes while addressing the systemic overmedicalization of childbirth in the U.S.

## Midwifery's Role in Underserved Areas

In rural or underserved areas, midwives play a particularly vital role, often serving as the primary healthcare providers for pregnant women. Here, midwives' ability to handle routine births and manage early-stage complications is critical, especially where access to obstetricians may be limited. In these settings, midwives not only provide maternity care but also contribute significantly to public health efforts, offering services such as contraception, family planning, and education on maternal health.

Midwives have carved out an essential space within the healthcare system, offering a care model centered on empowering women, ensuring safety, and improving maternal health outcomes. Their presence in hospitals, birth centers, and homes reflects the profession's adaptability and ability to meet diverse healthcare needs.

# Chapter 3

# Significance of ACOG and ACNM Guidelines

---

The American College of Obstetricians and Gynecologists (ACOG) and the American College of Nurse-Midwives (ACNM) provide essential guidelines that shape and define the practices of midwifery in the U.S. These guidelines are critical in ensuring that midwives deliver care that is evidence-based, safe, and aligned with the latest medical research and public health standards. Together, they create a balanced framework that integrates midwifery into the broader healthcare system while preserving midwives' distinct approach to maternal care.

## ACOG: Setting Medical Standards for Maternity Care

As the leading professional association for obstetricians and gynecologists, ACOG plays a key role in setting clinical standards for maternity care. Although ACOG primarily serves physicians, its guidelines on maternity care, such as those related to labor management, fetal monitoring, and the use of interventions like cesarean sections, are crucial for midwives as well. For midwives practicing in hospitals, adherence to ACOG guidelines ensures that their practices are consistent with those of their physician colleagues, fostering better collaboration and integration within healthcare teams.

ACOG also recognizes the value of midwifery in improving maternal outcomes, advocating for collaborative care models where midwives and obstetricians work together to ensure optimal patient outcomes.

## ACNM: Defining the Midwifery Model of Care

ACNM, as the leading organization for midwifery, offers a more midwife-centered set of guidelines that focus on the unique competencies and skills midwives bring to maternal care. ACNM guidelines emphasize the midwifery model of care, which prioritizes:

- Natural childbirth and minimal intervention.
- Patient-centered care that respects women's autonomy in healthcare decisions.
- Holistic support addressing the cultural, emotional, and psychological aspects of childbirth.

ACNM's standards of practice also ensure that midwives stay current with continuing education, licensing requirements, and adherence to ethical standards that promote patient safety and well-being.

## ACOG and ACNM: A Collaborative Approach

The synergy between ACOG and ACNM guidelines creates a balanced framework for midwifery practice. While ACOG offers protocols grounded in medical safety, ACNM emphasizes the midwife's role in providing holistic, woman-centered care. These guidelines ensure that midwives can work collaboratively with physicians when necessary while maintaining their distinct approach to pregnancy and childbirth. The collaboration between these two organizations exemplifies the shared goal of improving maternal health outcomes and ensuring that women receive the best possible care, regardless of their choice of birth provider. In sum, ACOG and ACNM guidelines form the backbone of professional midwifery practice in the United States, providing a solid foundation for midwives to offer safe, evidence-based, and compassionate care.

**Regulation of Licensed Midwives (LMs), Certified Midwives (CMs), and Certified Professional Midwives (CPMs)**

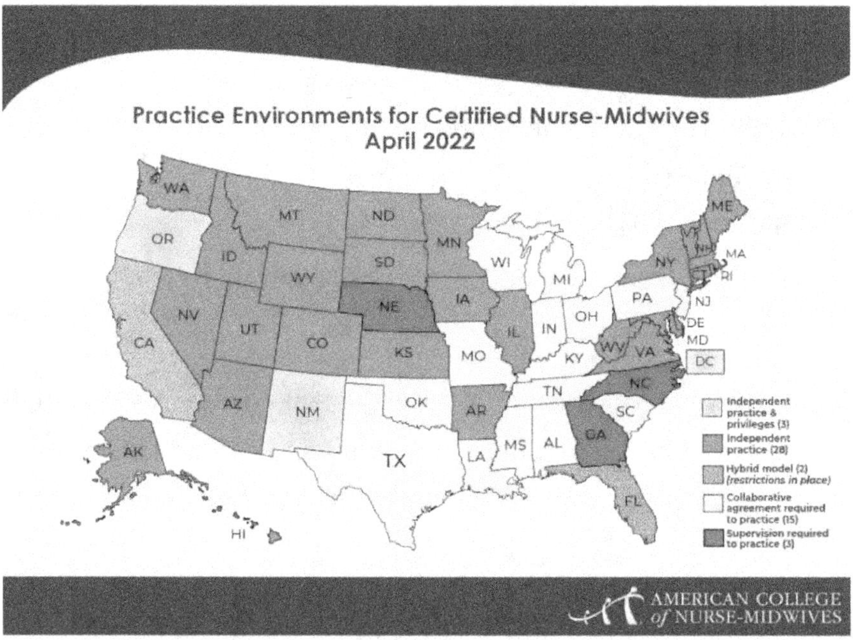


Licensed Midwives (LMs), Certified Midwives (CMs), and Certified Professional Midwives (CPMs) hold respected positions within their communities, offering valuable care to families seeking midwifery services, particularly in home and birth center settings. However, unlike Certified Nurse-Midwives (CNMs), these providers do not operate under the direct oversight of organizations such as the American College of Obstetricians and Gynecologists (ACOG) or the

American College of Nurse-Midwives (ACNM). Instead, their licensure, regulation, and clinical practice are governed by state-specific regulatory boards or agencies and peer review processes within their professional networks.

The decentralized nature of their regulation can lead to variability in standards of care, depending on the state's requirements for education, certification, and practice oversight. Some states have robust regulatory frameworks that ensure high competency levels, requiring comprehensive training, national certification, and continuing education for LMs, CMs, and CPMs. In these contexts, safety and adherence to evidence-based practices are well-maintained. However, the probability of mismanagement or deviations from standard care may increase in states with less stringent regulations or no formal licensing requirements for midwives. This variability raises concerns about accountability and consistency in the quality of care provided.

## The Role of Peer Review and Professional Networks

Peer review and collaborative interactions within midwifery are important in maintaining professional standards among LMs, CMs, and CPMs. These processes provide case evaluations, knowledge sharing, and professional development opportunities. While these peer-led initiatives are valuable, they may lack the robust oversight mechanisms present in hospital-based systems or organizations like ACNM, which provide structured pathways for accountability and remediation.

Despite these challenges, the goal for all midwives (LMs, CMs, and CPMs) should be to prioritize patient safety and adhere to evidence-based practices, particularly when serving low-risk populations. However, the potential for adverse outcomes may be heightened when complications arise that require advanced medical interventions or hospital transfers. This underscores the importance of clear communication and collaborative relationships between community midwives and obstetric providers to ensure seamless care transitions when needed.

Efforts to standardize midwives' education, certification, and regulation across all states could further enhance safety and trust in midwifery care. By bridging the gaps between various midwifery certifications and fostering stronger connections with medical systems, the profession as a whole could mitigate risks and continue to provide high-quality, patient-centered care in all settings.

# Chapter 4

# Scope of Practice and Autonomy of Midwives

---

The autonomy of midwives is a cornerstone of their role in the healthcare system, particularly for Certified Nurse Midwives (CNMs), who are recognized as primary care providers for women. CNMs are highly trained professionals with the authority to manage low-risk pregnancies, labor, and postpartum care independently, making critical decisions for their patients without the need for direct oversight from physicians. This autonomy allows midwives to offer care that is deeply personal, holistic, and centered on the woman's unique needs while also ensuring the safety and well-being of both mother and baby.

At the heart of midwifery autonomy is the philosophy of woman-centered care, which views pregnancy and childbirth as natural life processes, not medical conditions requiring routine intervention. Midwives, especially CNMs, are trained to provide individualized care that respects each woman's preferences, empowering them to make informed decisions about their health. This autonomy extends beyond childbirth, as midwives often provide a wide range of services, including family planning, reproductive health care, and routine gynecological exams. The autonomy of midwives is critical in both hospital and out-of-hospital settings, allowing them to adapt their care to different environments while maintaining the highest standards of practice.

## Defined Scope of Midwifery Care and Responsibilities

CNMs provide comprehensive care for women from adolescence through menopause, with a focus on reproductive health. In addition to prenatal and postnatal care, they perform routine gynecological exams, have full prescriptive authority, provide contraception counseling, and manage menopause-related care. During pregnancy, their responsibilities include monitoring the health of both the mother and the baby, offering guidance on prenatal nutrition and lifestyle, conducting routine tests, and preparing women for labor and delivery. Midwives also play a critical role in educating and supporting women, helping them make informed choices about their care.

During labor and delivery, CNMs focus on supporting the natural birthing process. They are skilled in managing normal, uncomplicated deliveries and are trained to intervene when necessary, such as administering medications, performing sutures, and managing postpartum hemorrhages. However, midwives work within a collaborative care framework, meaning they consult with or refer patients to obstetricians or other specialists when complications arise that are beyond their scope of practice. This ensures that patients receive the appropriate level of care while allowing CNMs to operate independently within their scope.

Postpartum midwives continue to support women by offering breastfeeding assistance, postpartum recovery care, and emotional support. They also monitor the health of newborns in the early stages and guide newborn care. This continuity of care is one of the hallmarks of midwifery practice, allowing midwives to build strong, trusting relationships with their patients.

AMERICAN COLLEGE *of* NURSE-MIDWIVES

## Comparison of Certified Nurse Midwives, Certified Midwives, and Certified Professional Midwives

*Clarifying the distinctions among professional midwifery credentials in the United States*

| | |
|---|---|
| International Confederation of Midwives' Definition of MIDWIFE | **While the profession of midwifery has developed differently in each country, we share a common understanding of the midwife internationally. The International Confederation of Midwives' definition is:**<br><br>The midwife is recognized as a responsible and accountable professional who works in partnership with women to give the necessary support, care and advice during pregnancy, labor, and the postpartum period, to conduct births on the midwife's own responsibility and to provide care for the newborn and the infant. This care includes preventative measures, the promotion of normal birth, the detection of complications in mother and child, the accessing of medical care or other appropriate assistance and the carrying out of emergency measures. The midwife has an important task in health counseling and education, not only for the woman, but also within the family and the community. This work should involve antenatal education and preparation for parenthood and may extend to women's health, sexual or reproductive health and childcare. A midwife may practice in any setting including the home, community, hospitals, clinics, or health units. |

| NATIONAL MIDWIFERY CREDENTIALS IN THE UNITED STATES OF AMERICA | CERTIFIED NURSE-MIDWIFE (CNM) | CERTIFIED MIDWIFE (CM) | CERTIFIED PROFESSIONAL MIDWIFE (CPM) |
|---|---|---|---|
| **EDUCATION** | | | |
| Minimum Degree Required for Certification | Graduate Degree | | Certification does not require an academic degree but is based on demonstrated competency in specified areas of knowledge and skills. |
| Minimum Education Requirements for Admission to Midwifery Education Program | Bachelor's Degree or higher from an accredited college or university AND | | High School Diploma or equivalent |
| | Earn RN license prior to or within midwifery education program. | Successful completion of required science & health courses and related health skills training prior to or within midwifery education program. | Prerequisites for accredited programs vary, but typically include specific courses such as statistics, microbiology, anatomy and physiology, and experience such as childbirth education or doula certification.<br><br>There are no specified requirements for entry to the North American Registry of Midwives (NARM) Portfolio Evaluation Process (PEP) pathway: an apprenticeship process that includes verification of knowledge and skills by qualified preceptors. |
| Clinical Experience Requirements | Attainment of knowledge, skills, and professional behaviors as identified by the American College of Nurse-Midwives (ACNM) Core Competencies for Basic Midwifery Education. | | Attainment of knowledge and skills, identified in the periodic job analysis conducted by NARM. |
| | Clinical education must occur under the supervision of an American Midwifery Certification Board (AMCB)-certified CNM/CM or other qualified preceptor who holds a graduate degree, has preparation for clinical teaching, and has clinical expertise and didactic knowledge commensurate with the content taught; >50% of clinical education must be under CNM/CM supervision. | | NARM requires that the clinical component of the educational process must be at least two years in duration and include a minimum of 55 births in three distinct categories. Clinical education must occur under the supervision of a midwife who must be nationally certified, legally recognized and who has practiced for at least three years and attended 50 out-of-hospital births post certification.<br><br>CPMs certified via the PEP may earn a Midwifery Bridge Certificate (MBC) to demonstrate they meet the International Confederation of Midwives (ICM) standards for minimum education. |
| **EDUCATION PROGRAM ACCREDITING ORGANIZATION** | | | |
| | The Accreditation Commission for Midwifery Education (ACME) is authorized by the U.S. Department of Education to accredit midwifery education programs and institutions. Midwifery education programs must be located within or affiliated with a regionally accredited institution. | | The Midwifery Education Accreditation Council (MEAC) is authorized by the U.S. Department of Education to accredit midwifery education programs and institutions. The scope of recognition includes certificate and degree-granting institutions, programs within accredited institutions, and distance education programs. |
| **SCOPE OF PRACTICE** | | | |
| Range of care provided | Midwifery as practiced by CNMs and CMs encompasses the independent provision of care during pregnancy, childbirth, and the postpartum period; sexual and reproductive health; gynecologic health; and family planning services, including preconception care. Midwives also provide primary care for individuals from adolescence throughout the lifespan as well as care for the healthy newborn during the first 28 days of life. Midwives provide care for all individuals who seek midwifery care, inclusive of all gender identities and sexual orientations.<br><br>CNMs/CMs provide initial and ongoing comprehensive assessment, diagnosis, and treatment. They conduct physical examinations; independently prescribe medications including but not limited to controlled substances, treatment of substance use disorder, and expedited partner therapy; admit, manage, and discharge patients; order and interpret laboratory and diagnostic tests; and order medical devices, durable medical equipment, and home health services.<br><br>Midwifery care as practiced by CNMs and CMs includes health promotion, disease prevention, risk assessment and management, and individualized wellness education and counseling. These services are provided in partnership with individuals and families in diverse settings such as ambulatory care clinics, private offices, telehealth and other methods of remote care delivery, community and public health systems, homes, hospitals, and birth centers. | | Midwifery as practiced by CPMs offers care, education, counseling and support to women and their families throughout the caregiving partnership, including pregnancy, birth and the postpartum period. CPMs provide on-going care throughout pregnancy and continuous, hands-on care during labor, birth and the immediate postpartum period, as well as maternal and well-baby care through the 6-8 week postpartum period.<br><br>CPMs provide initial and ongoing comprehensive assessment, diagnosis, and treatment. CPMs are trained to recognize abnormal or dangerous conditions requiring consultation with and/or referral to other healthcare professionals. They conduct physical examinations, administer medications, and use devices as allowed by state law, order and interpret laboratory and diagnostic tests. |
| Practice Settings | All settings - hospitals, homes, birth centers, and offices. The majority of CNMs and CMs attend births in hospitals. | | Homes, birth centers, and offices. The majority of CPMs attend births in homes and/or birth centers. |

| | | | |
|---|---|---|---|
| Prescriptive Authority | All US jurisdictions | Maine, Maryland, New York, Rhode Island, Virginia, and Washington, DC | CPMs do not maintain prescriptive authority; however, they may obtain and administer certain medications in select states. |
| Third Party Reimbursement | Most private insurance; Medicaid coverage mandated in all states; Medicare, TRICARE | Most private insurance; Medicaid coverage in Maine, Maryland, New York, Rhode Island, and Washington, DC | Private insurance mandated in 6 states; coverage varies in other states; 13 states include CPMs in state Medicaid plans |
| **CERTIFICATION** | | | |
| NATIONAL MIDWIFERY CREDENTIALS IN THE UNITED STATES OF AMERICA | CERTIFIED NURSE-MIDWIFE (CNM) | CERTIFIED MIDWIFE (CM) | CERTIFIED PROFESSIONAL MIDWIFE (CPM) |
| Certifying Organization | American Midwifery Certification Board (AMCB) | | North American Registry of Midwives (NARM) |
| | AMCB and NARM are accredited by the National Commission for Certifying Agencies | | |
| Requirements Prior to Taking National Certification Exam | Graduation from a midwifery education program accredited by the Accreditation Commission for Midwifery Education (ACME);<br>AND<br>Verification by program director of completion of education program<br>AND<br>Verification of master's degree or higher<br><br>**CNMs must also submit evidence of an active RN license at time of initial certification* | | Graduation from a midwifery education program accredited by the Midwifery Education Accreditation Council (MEAC)<br>OR<br>Completion of NARM's Portfolio Evaluation Process (PEP)<br>OR<br>AMCB-Certified CNM/CM with at least ten community-based birth experiences<br>OR<br>Completion of an equivalent state licensure program<br><br>All applicants must also submit evidence of current adult CPR and neonatal resuscitation certification or course completion |
| Recertification Requirement | Every 5 years | | Every 3 years |
| **LICENSURE** | | | |
| Legal Status | Licensed in 50 states plus the District of Columbia and U.S. territories as midwives, nurse-midwives, advanced practice registered nurses, or nurse practitioners. | Licensed in Arkansas, Colorado, Delaware, Hawaii, Maine, Maryland, New Jersey, New York, Oklahoma, Rhode Island, Virginia, and the District of Columbia. | Licensed in 37 states and the District of Columbia. |
| Licensure Agency | Boards of Midwifery, Medicine, Nursing or Departments of Health | Boards of Midwifery, Medicine, Nursing, Complementary Health Care Providers or Departments of Health | Boards of Midwifery, Medicine, Nursing, Complementary Health Care Providers; Departments of Health or Departments of Professional Licensure or Regulation |
| **PROFESSIONAL ASSOCIATION** | | | |
| | American College of Nurse-Midwives (ACNM | | National Association of Certified Professional Midwives (NACPM) |
| *Note: This document does not address individuals who are not certified and may attend births with or without legal recognition.* | | | |

*Updated: ACNM Government Affairs | May 2023*

# Chapter 5

# Comparison of Midwifery Care vs. Obstetrical Care

Midwifery and obstetrical care differ in both philosophy and practice. While both prioritize safe, effective care for women and babies, midwifery follows a holistic, patient-centered approach, whereas obstetrics is more medicalized, focusing on managing potential complications through intervention.

Midwives view childbirth as a natural process that typically requires minimal medical intervention. They promote position changes during labor—such as squatting, hands and knees, or side-lying—to facilitate fetal alignment, optimize pelvic space, and enhance uterine contractions, reducing the need for interventions.

Obstetricians, skilled in managing complications, often employ continuous fetal monitoring, intravenous fluids, epidurals, and labor augmentation with oxytocin. While these interventions are essential in certain cases, they can limit movement and hinder natural labor progression.

Midwifery emphasizes continuous support throughout labor, which is linked to lower intervention rates and higher maternal satisfaction. Obstetricians who are managing multiple patients may be present primarily during active labor or complications.

However, midwifery and obstetrics are not mutually exclusive. In many healthcare settings, they collaborate—midwives handling low-risk births while obstetricians address complications—ensuring individualized, comprehensive care.

## Benefits of Midwife-Led Care Models: Less Intervention, Holistic Focus

Midwifery care reduces unnecessary interventions while fostering a holistic approach to childbirth. Research shows women receiving midwife-led care experience lower rates of cesarean sections, episiotomies, and labor inductions. A Cochrane Database review found midwifery care decreased cesarean rates by 24% and episiotomies by 16%. The Lancet reported midwifery care lowered labor induction rates by 21%, improving outcomes for mothers and babies.

Midwives prioritize the natural progression of labor and use non-invasive techniques such as hydrotherapy, massage, breathing exercises, and position changes for pain management. Their emphasis on emotional and physical well-being fosters a supportive birth environment, leading to positive experiences and better outcomes.

Midwife-led care also enhances maternal satisfaction. Women report feeling more supported and involved in decision-making due to midwives' patient-centered approach. Their focus on autonomy and collaboration with physicians, when needed, ensures women receive appropriate care tailored to their needs.

In summary, midwifery promotes natural childbirth, reduces unnecessary interventions, and prioritizes holistic well-being. Its emphasis on personalized, continuous support results in better outcomes and greater satisfaction for birthing individuals.

**Birth Objectives By Provider**

| Subject/Item | LPM/CPM | CNM | Private practice MD | Academic MD | corporate MD | HospitalistMD |
|---|---|---|---|---|---|---|
| safe baby | xx | xxx | xxxx | xxxx | xxxx | xxxx |
| safe mom | xxx | xxxx | xxxx | xxx | xxxx | xxxx |
| maternal fetal connection | xxx | xxx | xx | xx | x | |
| mind and body healing | xxx | xxxx | xx | x | | |
| autonomy | xxx | xxxx | xx | x | | |
| PTSD and trauma | xxx | xxx | x | | | |
| empowering women | xxx | xxxx | x | | | |

# Chapter 6

# Collaboration in Hospital Settings: The Need for CNM-Physician Collaboration in Teaching Hospitals

Collaboration between Certified Nurse Midwives (CNMs) and physicians is critical in hospital settings, particularly in teaching hospitals where multiple levels of care providers interact. The dynamic environment of a teaching hospital offers a unique opportunity for CNMs, obstetricians (OBs), and residents to work together to optimize patient care, create learning opportunities, and strengthen healthcare delivery. In such institutions, collaboration is not just a matter of convenience but a necessity for patient safety and improved outcomes.

The need for collaboration in teaching hospitals arises from the complexity and diversity of cases handled within these facilities. While midwives are equipped to manage normal, low-risk pregnancies and births, teaching hospitals often handle a mix of routine and high-risk cases. In high-risk situations, CNMs must collaborate with physicians, such as OB-GYNs and Maternal-Fetal Medicine (MFM) specialists, to ensure that patients receive appropriate care. Effective collaboration allows for smooth transitions when complications arise, ensuring that both mother and baby are cared for by the right provider at the right time.

Moreover, the presence of medical residents introduces another layer of complexity. Residents are still in the learning phase of their careers and often require guidance from both attending physicians and CNMs.

In this context, CNMs are crucial in mentoring and guiding residents in midwifery-led care practices, ensuring that residents understand the importance of non-interventionist strategies and holistic care. Collaboration, therefore, becomes a two-way street: CNMs benefit from the support and expertise of physicians in high-risk cases, while physicians and residents gain valuable insights into the midwifery model of care.

Collaboration between CNMs and physicians in teaching hospitals is also vital for creating a comprehensive learning environment. Both OBs and CNMs bring unique strengths to the table: while OBs have expertise in surgical interventions and management of complications, CNMs excel in supporting natural birth and minimizing interventions. By working together, they can offer a well-rounded approach to maternity care that embraces the best of both fields and ensures the patient's needs are prioritized.

CNM-physician collaboration in teaching hospitals promotes a culture of mutual respect, continuous learning, and patient-centered care. It ensures that each provider operates at the highest level of their training while maintaining flexibility in responding to the needs of individual patients. By combining the strengths of midwifery and obstetrics, teaching hospitals can set an example for collaborative practice that benefits healthcare providers and patients.

## Clear Role Delineation Between CNMs, OB Residents, and Attending Physicians

Effective collaboration requires clear role delineation between Certified Nurse Midwives (CNMs), OB residents, and attending physicians. Each professional plays a distinct role in maternity care, and ensuring these roles are well-defined is critical for seamless patient management, especially in high-stakes environments like teaching hospitals.

CNMs are autonomous practitioners trained to handle normal, low-risk pregnancies and deliveries. In hospitals, they are often the primary care providers for women experiencing uncomplicated pregnancies. CNMs conduct prenatal visits, manage labor and delivery, and provide postpartum care. Their approach is grounded in supporting the natural process of birth, emphasizing minimizing unnecessary interventions. CNMs consult or collaborate with physicians only when complications arise, such as the need for a cesarean section, assisted vaginal deliveries, or when managing high-risk conditions like uncontrolled gestational diabetes or severe preeclampsia.

OB residents, on the other hand, are still in training and work under the supervision of attending physicians. Their role involves learning to manage a broad range of obstetric scenarios, from routine deliveries to complex, high-risk cases. Residents often rotate through various areas of obstetrics, and during their rotations in labor and delivery, they collaborate closely with both CNMs and attending OB-GYNs. While residents are expected to gain hands-on experience, they must also respect the established patient-care relationship that CNMs have built with their patients. Residents must recognize the scope of practice of midwives, consulting them on decisions related to routine births and deferring to their expertise in normal labor and delivery scenarios.

Attending physicians serve as the highest authority in the hospital setting and are responsible for overseeing both residents and CNMs. In teaching hospitals, they play a key role in supervising the care provided by residents and stepping in during complicated or high-risk cases.

While attending physicians have extensive experience in managing high-risk pregnancies and performing surgical interventions, their role in routine deliveries is often limited unless a complication occurs. In collaborative care models, attending physicians respect the autonomy of CNMs, stepping in when needed and requested without undermining the midwife's role as the primary caregiver in low-risk cases.

Clear role delineation ensures that there is no overlap or confusion regarding who is responsible for specific aspects of care. This delineation fosters mutual respect among CNMs, OB residents, and attending physicians, ensuring that each provider can focus on their strengths while collaborating effectively for the best outcomes. In practice, this means that CNMs manage normal deliveries, consult with OB residents when needed, and escalate care to attending physicians in high-risk situations or emergencies.

OB residents, in turn, support CNMs and attending physicians, gaining valuable experience while respecting midwives' scope of practice. Attending physicians provide oversight and intervention when necessary, ensuring that all patients receive the necessary care.

## Effective Communication Strategies to Preserve Midwife Autonomy

Effective communication is key to preserving the autonomy of CNMs while fostering collaboration with physicians and residents in hospital settings. In many cases, poor communication can lead to misunderstandings about roles and responsibilities, potentially undermining the midwife's position as the primary care provider. To prevent this, hospitals must establish clear communication protocols that promote transparency, respect, and teamwork.

One of the most important strategies for maintaining clear communication is the pre-conference or pre-briefing session conducted in an SBAR format. SBAR—an acronym for Situation, Background, Assessment, and Recommendation—is a standardized communication tool that ensures concise, focused, and efficient information exchange, especially in high-stakes environments like healthcare.

Before entering a patient's room, the midwife and physician should engage in a brief SBAR-based discussion to clarify the situation, outline their respective roles, and align on a collaborative approach:

1. **Situation:** The midwife begins by describing the immediate situation or concern. For example, *"The patient is in active*

*labor, currently dilated to 6cm, with contractions occurring every three minutes."*

2. **Background:** The midwife provides relevant background information, such as the patient's medical history, birth preferences, or any complications observed during prenatal care. This helps the physician understand the patient's context. For instance, *"She has a history of rapid labor and prefers minimal intervention."*

3. **Assessment:** The midwife shares their clinical assessment of the current situation, offering professional observations and insights. For example, *"Her vital signs are stable, and both maternal and fetal monitoring show no signs of distress. However, the patient has expressed concerns about pain management."*

4. **Recommendation:** Finally, the midwife recommends the next steps, ensuring both parties have input. For example, *"I recommend allowing her to continue laboring in the tub for pain relief, with intermittent monitoring for the next hour. What are your thoughts?"*

Using SBAR ensures that communication remains organized, avoids unnecessary details, and prioritizes actionable information. This framework fosters mutual understanding and collaboration, ensuring the physician has the context needed to support the patient without undermining the midwife's established relationship. Furthermore, it enhances patient-centered care by integrating the midwife's insights into decision-making.

By adopting SBAR during pre-briefings, the midwife and physician can seamlessly coordinate their efforts, reinforcing trust and respect while focusing on the patient's well-being.

Once inside the patient's room, the midwife must introduce the physician to the patient, preserving the trust and rapport that has been established throughout the course of care. This introduction should be warm and professional and affirm the collaborative nature of their roles. For example, the midwife might say, *"This is Dr. (Last Name), who is here to assist us and ensure everything continues smoothly. I'll remain with you throughout, and together, we'll support you in achieving the birth plan you've envisioned."*

This approach communicates to the patient that the physician is there to assist rather than take over, fostering a sense of continuity and respect in the patient's care experience. By maintaining the midwife's established leadership and involvement, the patient is reassured that her preferences and birth plan remain central to the process.

Additionally, it is imperative to secure the patient's informed consent before inviting a new provider into her birth space. This involves explaining the reason for the physician's presence, addressing any concerns the patient may have, and ensuring she understands her options. For instance, the midwife might say, *"I'd like to introduce Dr. (Last Name), who can provide additional expertise if needed. Are you comfortable having them join us to discuss how we can best support you briefly?"*

In collaborative care settings, such introductions are more than a formality—they are a critical step in maintaining the patient's autonomy and confidence. This process reinforces the idea that the patient is active in her care, ensuring she feels respected and empowered during this pivotal experience.

Another effective communication strategy involves shared decision-making. When a physician's input is required, the midwife and physician should collaborate in real time to discuss the best course of action. This means involving the patient in the decision-making process, explaining the rationale behind any proposed interventions, and ensuring that the patient's preferences are considered. By maintaining open, respectful dialogue, midwives can assert their autonomy while benefiting from the physician's expertise.

Hospitals should implement debriefing sessions after complex or high-risk cases as a standard practice. These sessions provide a structured opportunity for certified nurse-midwives (CNMs), residents, physicians (OB, Anesthesia, and Neonatal), and registered nurses to reflect on the care provided, evaluate outcomes, and address any challenges encountered. Such discussions enable team members to identify successes, explore areas for improvement, and share valuable insights from different professional perspectives. By fostering an environment of open dialogue, regular debriefings promote a culture of continuous learning, enhance team cohesion, and help resolve any communication breakdowns that may have arisen during care delivery. Additionally, these sessions serve to emphasize the integral role of midwifery care within the broader maternity care team, reinforcing mutual respect and collaboration.

To further enhance communication and collaboration, hospitals should adopt standardized communication tools such as structured handoffs or frameworks like SBAR (Situation, Background, Assessment, Recommendation). These tools help streamline the transfer of critical information between midwives, physicians, and residents, ensuring that all parties are aligned in their understanding of the patient's condition and care plan.

The use of such frameworks reduces the risk of miscommunication, minimizes omissions, and ensures clarity during transitions or collaborative interventions. This is especially important during high-stakes situations, where timely and accurate information can significantly impact outcomes.

By integrating these strategies into hospital workflows, facilities can improve teamwork and communication while preserving the autonomy and clinical expertise of CNMs in managing patient care. This balance is essential for providing patient-centered, high-quality maternity care that respects the unique strengths of each team member.

## High-Risk Management and Collaboration

Managing high-risk pregnancies and deliveries requires seamless collaboration between Certified Nurse-Midwives (CNMs) and obstetricians (OB-GYNs). While CNMs are highly skilled in managing low-risk pregnancies autonomously, the complexities of high-risk cases demand a multidisciplinary approach to ensure optimal outcomes for both mother and baby.

In high-risk scenarios—such as pregnancies affected by preeclampsia, gestational diabetes, preterm labor, or multiple gestations—early identification of risk factors is paramount. CNMs are trained to recognize when a pregnancy falls outside their scope of practice or comfort level. Midwives collaborate with OB-GYNs to create a detailed, individualized care plan when such risk factors are identified. This may include closer monitoring, advanced diagnostic testing, pharmacological management, or planning for surgical interventions, such as cesarean delivery, if necessary.

The collaborative relationship between CNMs and physicians becomes particularly vital during labor and delivery. For example:

- **Fetal Distress:** A CNM initiates fetal monitoring, repositions the mother, and provides oxygen while consulting with an OB-GYN for additional interventions like expedited delivery.
- **Shoulder Dystocia:** The midwife employs maneuvers to resolve the dystocia, while the physician is prepared to escalate care if the initial techniques are ineffective.
- **Postpartum Hemorrhage:** The CNM initiates measures like uterine massage and medication administration while coordinating with the physician for surgical or more advanced interventions if needed.

These examples underscore how midwives and physicians can effectively share responsibilities, ensuring that care escalates smoothly without compromising the patient's safety or the midwife's role as the primary caregiver.

To support effective collaboration, hospitals should establish clear escalation protocols. These protocols should:

1. Define the criteria for when care transitions from midwife-led to physician-led management.

2. Clarify roles and responsibilities during emergencies to prevent confusion.
3. Promote proactive communication, ensuring that all providers are aware of the patient's status and care plan.

Such protocols minimize delays in care, streamline decision-making, and enhance teamwork, creating an environment where CNMs and OB-GYNs can effectively contribute their expertise.

By combining the patient-centered, holistic approach of midwifery care with the advanced medical knowledge of obstetricians, collaborative high-risk management ensures that every patient receives the best of both worlds. This partnership balances the midwifery model's emphasis on natural processes with the ability to address complications decisively, ultimately leading to safer and more personalized maternity care.

# Chapter 7

## The Role of Midwives in Collaborative Care, Assisted Delivery and C-Sections

During assisted deliveries and cesarean sections (C-sections), collaboration between Certified Nurse Midwives (CNMs) and obstetricians is crucial to ensure safe and effective care. CNMs, though skilled in handling routine vaginal deliveries, are also integral to the collaborative care process when interventions like forceps delivery, vacuum extraction, or C-sections become necessary. In these situations, CNMs work alongside obstetricians to maintain the continuity of care and ensure that their patients receive medical expertise and emotional support.

### Training and Competency Requirements

For a CNM to perform assisted vaginal deliveries, rigorous training is essential. This training typically involves:

- **Didactic Education:** Gaining an in-depth understanding of the indications, risks, and techniques associated with vacuum and forceps delivery.
- **Simulation Training:** Practicing procedures in a controlled, simulated environment to develop technical proficiency.

- **Clinical Oversight:** These deliveries are performed under the direct supervision of an experienced physician until the CNM demonstrates consistent competency.

This layered approach ensures that CNMs are well-equipped to perform these procedures safely and effectively while maintaining a collaborative relationship with the supervising physician.

## State-Specific Scope of Practice Regulations

The ability of CNMs to perform assisted vaginal deliveries is governed by state laws, which define their scope of practice. For example:

- **Permissive States:** In some states, CNMs are explicitly allowed to perform assisted vaginal deliveries as long as they adhere to training and supervision requirements. These states often have robust midwifery practice acts that recognize the advanced skills of CNMs.

- **Restrictive States:** Other states may limit the scope of practice, requiring all assisted vaginal deliveries to be performed exclusively by physicians, regardless of the CNM's training or experience.

Hospitals and healthcare systems further define policies that may expand or restrict CNM practices within the framework of state laws.

## Legality in Dire Emergencies

In emergencies requiring immediate action to save the mother or baby's life, legal principles such as the *"Good Samaritan"* laws or the doctrine of necessity may protect CNMs from performing procedures outside their standard scope of practice. For example:

- **Good Samaritan Laws:** In some jurisdictions, these laws shield healthcare providers from liability when they act in good faith during emergencies, even if the action exceeds their usual scope.
- **Doctrine of Necessity:** This legal principle recognizes that lifesaving measures may be taken in emergencies when delay could result in harm or death.

However, these protections typically apply only in dire situations where no other qualified practitioner is available, and the actions taken must be reasonable and aligned with the CNM's knowledge and training. Documentation of the circumstances and decision-making process is critical in such cases.

## Collaborative Approach to Assisted Deliveries and High-Risk Pregnancy Management

Even when authorized to perform assisted vaginal deliveries, CNMs operate within a collaborative framework. The supervising physician's presence ensures that advanced interventions or surgical options are immediately available if complications arise.

This collaboration benefits patients by providing a safety net while allowing the CNM to maintain continuity of care during labor and delivery.

## Benefits and Challenges

**Benefits:**

- Expanding CNM capabilities improves access to skilled providers, particularly in rural or underserved areas.
- Patients benefit from continuity of care and a less fragmented birth experience.
- Collaborative models strengthen interprofessional relationships, enhancing patient outcomes.

**Challenges:**

- Inconsistencies in state regulations can create confusion and limit the full utilization of CNMs' skills.
- Ensuring adequate training and ongoing competency assessments can be resource-intensive.

By navigating these complexities and advocating for clear policies, healthcare systems can better integrate CNMs into collaborative care models, maximizing their contributions while maintaining patient safety.

When a cesarean section becomes necessary, Certified Nurse-Midwives (CNMs) play crucial roles in ensuring that the patient receives holistic and patient-centered care. Their dual contributions as First Assist and Labor Support highlight their versatility and dedication to continuity of care.

## The Role of First Assist

As First Assist, CNMs actively participate in the surgical process, providing essential support to the obstetrician. This role involves:

- **Surgical Assistance:** Tasks such as suctioning, managing retractors, or providing hemostasis during the procedure.
- **Suturing:** In some cases, CNMs assist with closing the surgical incision, demonstrating their surgical expertise.
- **Monitoring:** Keeping a vigilant eye on the patient's vital signs and overall condition throughout the procedure.

By participating as First Assist, CNMs bring a unique perspective to the surgical team. Their familiarity with the patient's medical history, preferences, and birth plan allows them to act as an advocate, ensuring the patient's voice is represented even in the operating room.

## Labor Support During Cesarean Sections

CNMs also play a vital role in providing emotional and physical support to the patient before, during, and after the surgery:

- **Pre-Surgical Support:** Preparing the patient for surgery, explaining the procedure, and addressing any last-minute concerns to alleviate anxiety.
- **Intraoperative Reassurance:** Offering comfort by maintaining eye contact, holding the patient's hand, or narrating what's happening to keep her informed.

- **Post-Surgical Continuity:** Immediately after the procedure, CNMs help with skin-to-skin contact if feasible, supporting breastfeeding initiation, and ensuring the patient feels cared for during recovery.

## Preserving Continuity of Care

One of the most significant benefits of having a CNM involved in a cesarean section is the continuity of care they provide. Unlike traditional models where the patient may meet a new provider in the operating room, the CNM's presence bridges the gap between labor and delivery, maintaining a familiar and trusted connection. This continuity has been shown to:

- Enhance patient satisfaction.
- Reduce feelings of fear or isolation during surgery.
- Improve postpartum recovery and bonding experiences.

## The Importance of Collaboration

The involvement of CNMs in cesarean sections underscores the collaborative nature of modern maternity care. Obstetricians, anesthesiologists, nurses, and CNMs work together to meet the patient's technical and emotional needs. This teamwork benefits the patient and fosters mutual respect and shared learning among healthcare providers.

## Challenges and Opportunities

**Challenges:**

- Variability in hospital policies and state regulations regarding CNMs' roles as First Assist.
- Limited access to training programs in surgical assisting for CNMs in some regions.

### Opportunities:

- Offering more CNMs training in surgical skills can enhance their ability to participate in cesarean sections, particularly in underserved areas.
- Promoting policies that support CNMs in surgical roles helps improve maternal outcomes and patient satisfaction.

The collaboration between CNMs and obstetricians during assisted deliveries and C-sections allows for a seamless blend of medical expertise and holistic care. By working together, midwives and obstetricians ensure that patients receive the necessary interventions while benefiting from the personalized support midwives provide.

## Managing High-Risk Pregnancies with OB-GYN Collaboration

For pregnancies involving conditions like diabetes, hypertension, or advanced maternal age, CNMs and OB-GYNs work together to provide comprehensive care.

### Key Aspects of Collaboration:

- CNMs identify risk factors and consult OB-GYNs to adjust care plans.

- Regular team meetings ensure coordinated management of complex cases.
- During labor, CNMs provide patient-centered support, while OB-GYNs oversee medical interventions.

This approach balances holistic midwifery care with medical expertise, improving outcomes for both mother and baby.

# Chapter 8

## Transfers from Out-of-Hospital to Hospital Settings: Ensuring a *"Soft Landing"*

While many out-of-hospital births progress smoothly, there are occasions when medical complications necessitate a transfer to the hospital setting. Common reasons for transfer include pain management, the need for vacuum or forceps-assisted delivery, cesarean section, increased fetal monitoring, or maternal emergencies such as hemorrhage.

These scenarios highlight the critical importance of a well-coordinated collaboration between midwives and hospital-based obstetric care teams. When midwives and OBs work together seamlessly, patients experience what can be described as a *"soft landing"*—a transition that prioritizes safety, respects patient preferences, and minimizes the emotional distress often associated with unexpected changes in a birth plan.

### Why Midwife-OB Collaboration is Essential in Transfers

1. **Continuity of Care During Transfers:** Midwives often accompany patients to the hospital, serving as advocates and ensuring that the patient's medical history, birth plan, and preferences are communicated effectively to the hospital care

team. This continuity helps to maintain trust and reduce anxiety during what can be a stressful time.

2. **A Multidisciplinary Approach to Care:** In hospital settings, CNMs and OBs bring complementary strengths. CNMs emphasize low-intervention care and patient-centered support, while OBs provide the advanced medical expertise needed to manage complications. Together, they create a balanced approach that addresses both medical and emotional needs.

3. **Streamlined Decision-Making:** Clear communication and shared protocols between midwives and OBs ensure timely emergency interventions. For example, in the event of fetal distress, the midwife may focus on maternal positioning and oxygen delivery while the OB assesses the need for surgical intervention.

4. **Patient Experience and Emotional Support:** Transfers can be emotionally challenging for patients, particularly if they deviate from their desired birth plan. A collaborative approach ensures that the patient remains at the center of care, with midwives providing reassurance and OBs offering expert medical guidance.

5. **Enhanced Postpartum Recovery:** Collaboration extends beyond delivery, as CNMs and OBs work together to manage postpartum care. This holistic approach addresses physical recovery and ensures that patients receive emotional and psychological support, promoting a more positive birth experience overall.

By integrating the strengths of midwifery care with obstetric expertise, hospital transfers can be transformed from potentially overwhelming situations into coordinated, patient-centered experiences that prioritize safety and respect for individual preferences.

## Postpartum Care Collaboration: CNMs Providing Continuity of Care

CNMs play a crucial role in postpartum care, ensuring continuity of care for both mother and baby. Even after complex deliveries, CNMs monitor physical recovery and provide emotional support. Collaboration with OB-GYNs is essential, especially when complications arise, but midwives' holistic approach ensures that patients receive comprehensive care that addresses both medical and emotional well-being.

After a vaginal birth, CNMs monitor for complications such as hemorrhage and perineal trauma while also supporting bonding and breastfeeding initiation. In cases of severe lacerations or postpartum hemorrhage, midwives work alongside OB-GYNs to manage the situation while maintaining a comforting presence for the patient. For C-section patients, CNMs assist with pain management, mobility, and emotional support, helping the mother process her birth experience and easing the transition to postpartum life.

Midwives are particularly instrumental in addressing birth trauma by fostering a supportive, patient-centered environment. Through informed consent and respectful care, they help patients feel in control, reducing the likelihood of traumatic experiences. In the postpartum period, CNMs screen for emotional distress, provide mental health resources, and guide mothers through newborn care, ensuring a positive transition into parenthood. This trauma-informed approach prevents long-term psychological distress and strengthens maternal confidence.

Collaboration between CNMs and OB-GYNs extends into postpartum recovery, especially when complications such as infections or delayed healing occur. Midwives coordinate follow-ups and ensure that care remains integrated and patient-centered. By blending medical expertise with holistic, compassionate support, the midwifery model enhances maternal health outcomes and promotes a more empowering postpartum experience for families.

# Chapter 9

## Conflict Resolution in Collaborative Care

Effective collaboration between CNMs and physicians is crucial for providing high-quality maternity care. However, despite the shared goal of delivering safe and effective care, conflicts can arise in hospital settings due to differences in clinical philosophies, communication styles, and misunderstandings about roles and responsibilities. If not addressed promptly and constructively, these conflicts can negatively impact patient care and the working relationship between healthcare providers. Therefore, conflict resolution is essential to collaborative care, ensuring that CNMs and physicians can work together smoothly while respecting each other's expertise and scope of practice.

In a hospital's complex and ever-demanding environment, CNMs and physicians must navigate various challenges, particularly when managing cases that require a balance between midwifery-led care and medical intervention. By understanding the common sources of conflict and adopting practical conflict resolution strategies, healthcare teams can maintain a collaborative atmosphere that supports patient-centered care and promotes mutual respect. This section will explore the common sources of conflict in hospital settings, outline steps for conflict resolution between CNMs and physicians, and highlight the importance of teaching OB residents about midwifery practices and scope.

## Sources of Conflict and How to Address Common Conflicts in Hospital Settings

Conflict between CNMs and physicians often arises due to differing approaches to childbirth, varying expectations about care management, and the hierarchical structure within hospital settings. The most common sources of conflict include:

1. **Differences in Clinical Philosophy:** Midwives and obstetricians often have distinct perspectives on childbirth. Midwifery care is rooted in the belief that pregnancy and childbirth are natural processes that generally proceed without the need for medical intervention. Midwives prioritize low-intervention approaches, supporting natural labor and delivery whenever possible. In contrast, physicians, particularly obstetricians, are trained to anticipate and manage complications, which may lead to a more intervention-heavy approach. These differences in philosophy can create tension, particularly when physicians perceive midwives as not acting swiftly enough in situations they believe require medical intervention.
2. **Miscommunication or Lack of Communication:** Clear communication is vital for effective collaboration, yet communication breakdowns are among the most common causes of conflict in hospital settings. Misunderstandings can occur when there is no clear discussion about roles or when clinical decisions are made without consulting all care team members. For example, a physician may step in to take over a patient's care without first discussing the situation with the CNM, leading to feelings of undermining or distrust. Likewise,

if a CNM does not clearly communicate their patient's preferences or condition, the physician may act without fully understanding the context, resulting in frustration on both sides.

3. **Role Confusion and Scope of Practice:** Confusion or disagreement over roles and responsibilities is another significant source of conflict. In teaching hospitals, this can be particularly pronounced with the presence of OB residents, who may not fully understand the scope of practice of midwives. Residents might assume that physicians should always take over in complex situations, even when the CNM can fully manage the situation. This confusion can lead to unnecessary interventions, a breakdown in trust, and frustration for both the midwife and the patient.
4. **Time Pressure and High-Stress Environments:** Labor and delivery units are often high-stress environments, particularly when complications arise. In such settings, time pressure can exacerbate conflicts between CNMs and physicians. In an emergency, for example, a physician may feel the need to intervene quickly, potentially overriding the CNM's autonomy. These situations can create tension if the midwife feels that her expertise is being disregarded or if the physician believes the midwife is not acting quickly enough.

Recognizing these sources of conflict is the first step in developing strategies to address and resolve them. By acknowledging and respecting the different perspectives and roles that each provider brings to the care team, CNMs and physicians can work together more effectively and reduce the likelihood of conflict.

## Practical Steps for Conflict Resolution Between CNMs and Physicians

Addressing conflicts between CNMs and physicians requires a proactive, structured approach that prioritizes communication, respect, and teamwork. The following practical steps can help resolve conflicts and maintain a collaborative environment in hospital settings:

1. **Pre-Conference Meetings and Open Dialogue:** One of the most effective ways to prevent conflicts is to establish regular pre-conference meetings between CNMs, physicians, and other care team members before entering a patient's room. These meetings provide an opportunity to discuss the patient's condition, review the care plan, and clarify roles. By aligning on the approach to care beforehand, both the midwife and physician can enter the room with a unified strategy, reducing the chances of miscommunication or role confusion.

2. **Mutual Respect for Expertise and Autonomy:** Conflict often arises when one provider feels that their expertise or autonomy is being undermined. Both CNMs and physicians must acknowledge and respect each other's skills and contributions. Midwives should be recognized for their expertise in low-intervention, patient-centered care, while physicians should be valued for managing complications and providing medical interventions when necessary. Acknowledging these strengths fosters mutual respect and ensures that care decisions are based on the patient's best interests rather than professional hierarchies.

3. **Real-Time Conflict Resolution:** When conflicts arise, it is important to address them in real time rather than allowing frustration to build. If a disagreement occurs during a patient's care, the CNM and physician should step aside for a moment to discuss the situation privately. This allows them to clarify their positions, express any concerns, and come to a resolution without disrupting the patient's experience. Real-time conflict resolution ensures that disagreements are addressed promptly, preventing them from escalating into more significant issues.

4. **Debriefing After Critical Events:** Holding a debriefing session with the care team is beneficial after managing a complex or high-stress situation. During this session, CNMs, physicians, and other staff can reflect on what went well and what could be improved. These debriefings provide an opportunity for open communication and learning, helping to identify any underlying issues that may have contributed to the conflict. By discussing the event non-judgmentally and collaboratively, healthcare teams can learn from their experiences and improve their future interactions.

5. **Structured Conflict Resolution Protocols:** Many hospitals have formal conflict resolution protocols that outline the steps to be taken when conflicts arise. These protocols typically involve escalating the issue to a higher level if it cannot be resolved between the CNM and physician. For example, if a disagreement cannot be resolved through direct communication, the care team may involve a department head or supervisor to mediate the discussion. Having a clear, structured process in place helps ensure that conflicts are resolved fairly and efficiently.

6. **Maintaining Patient-Centered Focus:** Keeping the patient's needs at the center of the discussion is essential throughout any conflict resolution process. CNMs and physicians share the goal of providing the best possible care for their patients. By focusing on the patient's well-being, providers can find common ground and work through their differences to prioritize the patient's experience and outcomes.

These practical steps help create a collaborative environment where conflicts can be addressed constructively, allowing CNMs and physicians to continue working together effectively.

## Teaching OB Residents About Midwifery Practices and Scope

One of the most effective ways to reduce conflict in hospital settings is to ensure that OB residents are properly educated about midwifery practices and the scope of midwives' responsibilities. Many conflicts arise because residents, who are still in the learning phase of their careers, may not fully understand the midwifery model of care or the autonomy that CNMs hold within the healthcare team.

## Orientation and Training:

When new OB residents join a labor and delivery unit, it is essential to provide them with a comprehensive orientation that includes an introduction to midwifery practices. This orientation should cover the scope of CNM practice, the midwifery model of care, and the importance of collaboration between CNMs and physicians. By establishing these expectations early on, residents can better understand when to consult with a midwife, when to defer to their expertise, and when it is appropriate to escalate care.

## Mentorship and Shadowing:

Another effective teaching strategy is to pair OB residents with experienced CNMs for shadowing and mentorship opportunities. Residents can observe firsthand how midwives manage labor and delivery by working closely with midwives, emphasizing the importance of non-interventionist approaches and patient-centered care. This experience allows residents to appreciate the value of midwifery care and to understand how midwives can work alongside physicians to provide comprehensive care.

## Simulation Training and Joint Learning Opportunities:

Joint training sessions and simulations that involve both CNMs and OB residents can help foster collaboration and mutual understanding. For example, simulation exercises for managing labor, deliveries, and emergencies can help both providers practice working together in real-world scenarios. These exercises improve clinical skills and teach effective communication and teamwork in high-stress environments.

## Clear Communication Expectations:

OB residents should also be taught the importance of clear and respectful communication when working with CNMs. This includes consulting the midwife before making any changes to the care plan, seeking input on routine care decisions, and involving the CNM in discussions with the patient. Teaching residents to value the midwife's role in patient care fosters a more collaborative atmosphere and reduces the likelihood of misunderstandings or conflicts arising.

By educating OB residents about midwifery practices and scope, hospitals can reduce role confusion, enhance collaboration, and create a more supportive environment for both midwives and physicians. This education ensures that future physicians understand the importance of working with CNMs as equal partners in maternity care, ultimately leading to better patient outcomes and a more harmonious care environment.

## Patient-Centered Approach and Autonomy

The patient-centered approach is at the core of midwifery care, emphasizing respect for the autonomy and preferences of the woman. Midwifery care is grounded in the belief that pregnancy and childbirth are natural processes and that women should have the primary say in decisions about their bodies and the birth experience. By fostering a collaborative relationship between the patient and care providers, midwives empower women to take an active role in their healthcare, ensuring that their preferences, concerns, and cultural values are respected. This approach stands in contrast to more medicalized models, which often prioritize clinical outcomes over patient preferences.

Midwives play a pivotal role in empowering patients through comprehensive prenatal education, emphasizing the importance of informed decision-making throughout the pregnancy journey. They dedicate significant time to teaching about the physical and emotional changes during pregnancy, the stages of labor and birth, and the essentials of postpartum recovery. This education often includes discussions about pain management options, birth plans, newborn care, and breastfeeding support, ensuring patients feel confident and prepared for the experiences ahead. By fostering a collaborative environment, midwives encourage patients to ask questions, voice concerns, and explore their preferences, equipping them with the knowledge to make choices that align with their values and needs. This holistic approach enhances patient autonomy and promotes a sense of empowerment during the antepartum, intrapartum, and postpartum periods, creating a foundation for positive outcomes and lasting confidence in their ability to navigate parenthood.

## Bottom of Form

Midwives believe that every woman is the expert on her own body and should be given the tools and information to make decisions that align with her values. In practice, this means that midwives spend time discussing the patient's birth plan, listening to her concerns, and providing evidence-based information about the benefits and risks of different interventions.

Whether the patient prefers a natural, low-intervention birth or chooses certain medical interventions, the midwife's goal is to support her choices and create an environment where those preferences are respected.

## Shared Decision-Making in High-Risk Scenarios and Ensuring Continuous Patient Engagement During Collaboration

Shared decision-making is a collaborative process in which the healthcare provider and patient collaborate to make informed choices. In high-risk pregnancies, this approach is crucial as medical interventions may be necessary, but patient autonomy should still be respected. Even when deviations from the birth plan occur, involving the patient in decision-making fosters trust and ensures that her values remain central to her care.

Transparency is key in high-risk scenarios. Patients must receive evidence-based information about their condition, potential risks, and available options. While medical teams provide expert recommendations, shared decision-making ensures that patients remain active participants in their care. This approach helps patients feel more in control, even during unexpected complications and strengthens their trust in their providers.

Consistent communication is essential for patient engagement. Midwives and physicians should inform patients about labor progress, explain care decisions, and address concerns. Regular check-ins allow patients to adjust their birth plans as needed, reinforcing their role in the decision-making process.

The continuity of care provided by midwives further enhances patient engagement. Even in high-risk cases where physicians take a leading role, CNMs often remain the patient's primary point of contact, offering emotional and physical support. This ongoing presence fosters stability and ensures patient-centered care that balances medical necessity with respect for patient preferences.

# Chapter 10

# Education and Training

A key factor in ensuring effective collaboration between Certified Nurse Midwives (CNMs) and physicians is continuous education and training that fosters mutual understanding and respect between these professionals. Through structured educational programs, hospitals can promote teamwork and equip all providers with the necessary skills to deliver patient-centered, collaborative care.

This training is particularly critical in environments where CNMs and physicians, including OB residents, work together to manage labor and delivery. Enhancing collaboration through ongoing education improves clinical outcomes and reduces conflicts, stigmas, miscommunication, and role confusion in high-pressure situations.

Training programs focusing on collaboration are essential in preparing midwives and physicians to work together effectively, particularly in teaching hospitals where OB residents are still developing their skills. Simulation exercises, orientation programs, ongoing mentorship, and case reviews are powerful tools for fostering a collaborative culture.

These initiatives ensure that all care providers understand each other's roles and can coordinate seamlessly in managing routine and high-risk deliveries.

## Enhancing Collaboration Through Training

Simulation exercises have become a significant part of clinical education, particularly in teaching hospitals where interprofessional collaboration is essential. For CNMs and OB-GYNs, including residents, simulation-based training offers a controlled environment where they can practice working together in various labor and delivery scenarios, from routine births to complex, high-risk situations. These exercises are invaluable in fostering collaboration, enhancing communication, and allowing team members to practice responding to emergencies in a coordinated manner.

One of the most significant benefits of simulation exercises is that they help CNMs and physicians develop a shared mental model of how to approach different childbirth scenarios. For example, during simulated shoulder dystocia—a situation where the baby's shoulder becomes stuck during delivery—the midwife may initiate initial maneuvers to release the baby. At the same time, the physician prepares to assist if the situation escalates. In this exercise, the CNM and physician can practice working together, understanding when it is appropriate to escalate care, and communicating effectively throughout the process. This type of hands-on, scenario-based learning helps to clarify roles and fosters a sense of trust between midwives and physicians.

Simulation exercises also provide an opportunity to practice emergency response protocols, such as those for postpartum hemorrhage, eclampsia, or cord prolapse. These are high-pressure situations where timely, coordinated action is critical. By practicing these scenarios in a low-stakes environment, midwives and physicians can improve their ability to work together efficiently during emergencies. Simulation training highlights the importance of clear, respectful communication. It ensures that all providers feel empowered to contribute to decision-making while recognizing when to defer to their colleagues based on expertise.

In addition to technical skills, simulation exercises allow CNMs and physicians to practice non-technical skills crucial in a collaborative environment, such as teamwork, leadership, and conflict resolution. For example, a midwife may lead a simulated labor scenario, guiding the team through an expected delivery while the physician observes or assists.

In another scenario, the physician may take the lead in a complex cesarean section, with the midwife providing support. These exercises emphasize the fluidity of roles and demonstrate that collaboration does not mean one profession takes precedence over the other; rather, it is about bringing together different skill sets to ensure the best possible outcomes for the patient. By incorporating regular joint training sessions and simulations into hospital education programs, healthcare teams can continuously improve their collaborative practices, ensuring that midwives and physicians are prepared to work together in any situation.

## Orientation Programs for OB Residents on CNM Collaboration

Fostering collaboration between CNMs and physicians requires a comprehensive effort to address the misunderstandings and stigmas surrounding midwifery care. One key strategy is ensuring that obstetrics and gynecology (OB) residents still in training receive a thorough education on midwifery's scope, philosophy, and evidence-based practices. Many conflicts between OB residents and midwives arise not from intentional disregard but from a lack of understanding about midwives' role in patient care and their contributions to labor and delivery management. Orientation programs and collaborative training opportunities can help bridge this gap, promoting mutual respect and a shared commitment to patient-centered care.

Much of the stigma around midwifery is rooted in misconceptions about its safety, professionalism, and educational rigor. Midwifery, especially in rural settings or home birth scenarios, is often wrongly perceived as less safe or less regulated than hospital-based obstetric care, despite research confirming the safety of midwife-led care for low-risk pregnancies. Historical biases have contributed to these misconceptions, painting midwifery as outdated or inferior to medicalized obstetrics, often ignoring its holistic approach and its emphasis on personalized, evidence-based care. Critics may question the educational background of midwives, failing to recognize that many CNMs undergo rigorous training, including graduate-level education, clinical apprenticeships, and certification processes designed to prepare them for a wide range of clinical scenarios and interdisciplinary collaboration.

These misconceptions are particularly pronounced in rural areas, where midwifery care may be viewed skeptically due to limited healthcare resources and the assumption that midwives lack access to advanced medical technology. Similarly, home births are often stigmatized as inherently risky, even though planned home births attended by qualified midwives can provide a safe and supportive environment. Addressing these stigmas requires public education and greater integration of midwifery into healthcare systems, emphasizing the training, professionalism, and patient-centered philosophy that underpins midwifery care. By fostering understanding and collaboration, healthcare systems can maximize the strengths of both midwives and physicians, improving outcomes and creating a more inclusive approach to maternal and newborn care.

An effective orientation program should begin by introducing OB residents to the midwifery model of care. This model is grounded in the belief that pregnancy and childbirth are natural processes that can often proceed without medical intervention. OB residents, who are trained in a more medicalized approach to childbirth, may not be fully aware of the midwifery philosophy of minimal intervention and patient-centered care. By learning about this approach, residents can develop a deeper appreciation for midwives' unique role in managing low-risk pregnancies and supporting natural births.

Similar to understanding the philosophy of midwifery care, OB residents need to be educated about the scope of practice of CNMs. While midwives can manage normal, uncomplicated births, they also know when to escalate care to a physician if complications arise. Residents should be taught to trust midwives' clinical judgment and understand that CNMs are trained to recognize when medical intervention is necessary. Orientation programs should emphasize that collaboration is about shared responsibility and that both midwives and physicians play critical roles in ensuring safe and effective care.

A key component of the orientation program should also be communication training. OB residents must learn how to communicate effectively with midwives, particularly when making decisions about patient care. This involves respecting the midwife's established relationship with the patient and ensuring that all discussions about care are conducted collaboratively rather than hierarchically. For example, residents should be encouraged to ask for the CNM's input before making clinical decisions, particularly when the midwife has been managing the patient's care throughout labor. Teaching residents to involve midwives in decision-making fosters a culture of teamwork and respect.

Orientation programs should include shadowing opportunities, where OB residents observe CNMs during routine prenatal visits, labor management, and deliveries. By witnessing midwives in action, residents can better understand how midwifery care is delivered and how it differs from traditional obstetric care. These shadowing experiences help residents develop respect for the midwifery model and build trust with the midwives they will be working alongside throughout their residency.

## Ongoing Mentorship and Case Reviews to Foster Learning

Collaboration between CNMs and physicians is not a one-time event but an ongoing process that requires continuous learning and reflection. To foster a collaborative culture, hospitals should implement ongoing mentorship programs and regular case reviews that encourage both midwives and physicians to learn from each other's experiences.

Mentorship programs are an excellent way to ensure that new OB residents and CNMs have the opportunity to build strong working relationships. Pairing a resident with an experienced midwife allows the resident to observe how the midwife manages labor and delivery, particularly in cases where medical intervention is not required. Through mentorship, residents can learn about the midwifery model of care hands-on and better understand how to collaborate with midwives in real clinical settings. Likewise, CNMs can benefit from mentorship relationships with experienced OB-GYNs, gaining insights into managing high-risk pregnancies and complex cases.

Case reviews are another valuable tool for fostering collaboration and improving clinical outcomes. By reviewing complex or challenging cases, CNMs and physicians can reflect on what went well and what could have been improved. These reviews provide an opportunity to discuss the decision-making process, clarify roles, and identify areas where communication or collaboration could be enhanced. Joint case reviews promote transparency and trust, as both midwives and physicians can learn from each other's perspectives and experiences. They also serve as a forum for celebrating successes and reinforcing the importance of teamwork.

In birth work, there are inevitably times when less-than-favorable outcomes occur, underscoring the importance of a standardized case review process to evaluate care and identify opportunities for improvement. Most healthcare systems have formalized procedures for reviewing such cases. Still, for these processes to be effective, all involved—including midwives—must clearly understand how the reviews are conducted and their purpose. A collaborative, non-punitive approach fosters an environment where healthcare providers can openly discuss care plans, management decisions, and outcomes without fear of blame. Midwives play a critical role in these reviews, as their unique perspectives and expertise in patient-centered, holistic care often shed light on factors that might be overlooked.

During reviews, communicating clearly, responding to questions professionally, and providing educational insights are essential to fostering mutual understanding and promoting system-wide learning. By approaching case reviews as opportunities for growth and interdisciplinary collaboration, healthcare teams can improve patient outcomes, enhance trust among providers, and ensure that care remains evidence-based and centered on the needs of patients and families.

# Chapter 11

# Quality Improvement and Safety Initiatives

Ensuring the highest standards of care in maternity services requires a concerted focus on continuous quality improvement (CQI) and safety initiatives. Midwifery and obstetric teams must work together to create a culture of safety where ongoing evaluation, reflection, and improvement are embedded into everyday practice. By collaborating on quality improvement (QI) projects and safety protocols, CNMs and OB-GYNs can enhance patient outcomes, reduce medical errors, and create a more supportive and efficient healthcare environment.

In this section, we will explore how midwifery and OB-GYN teams can jointly contribute to CQI projects, the importance of safety protocols in managing high-risk pregnancies, and how feedback loops are essential in driving continuous improvement.

## Continuous Quality Improvement (CQI) and Safety: Joint Responsibility for QI Projects in Midwifery and OB-GYN

One of the most effective ways to improve the quality of maternity care is through collaboration between midwives and physicians on quality improvement (QI) projects. These projects identify areas where care can be enhanced, track outcomes, and implement changes that lead to better patient experiences and results. Continuous Quality Improvement involves a systematic approach to evaluating practices, developing new processes, and ensuring that healthcare providers consistently meet high standards of care.

CNMs and OB-GYNs share a joint responsibility for contributing to QI projects, as both professions bring unique perspectives and expertise. CNMs, with their focus on patient-centered care and natural childbirth, can offer valuable insights into reducing unnecessary interventions and improving patient satisfaction. OB-GYNs, who are experts in managing high-risk pregnancies and performing surgical interventions, bring critical knowledge about managing complications and improving maternal and fetal safety. By working together, these two groups can identify best practices that enhance care for all women, regardless of whether they are experiencing a routine or high-risk pregnancy.

A collaborative QI project might focus on reducing cesarean section rates in low-risk pregnancies, a common goal in maternity care. CNMs, who often support natural childbirth and minimal intervention, can contribute strategies for improving labor management practices to avoid unnecessary surgical interventions. OB-GYNs can provide guidance on how to safely balance these goals with the need to manage complications effectively when they arise. By developing shared protocols and consistently reviewing outcomes, both midwives and physicians can play an active role in achieving this goal.

Another area where joint QI projects are particularly beneficial is in the management of postpartum hemorrhage, a potentially life-threatening complication. Midwives and physicians can collaborate on developing and implementing protocols to quickly identify and manage this condition, with each provider bringing their expertise. Midwives may focus on early detection and initial management, while OB-GYNs may provide input on surgical interventions and medical management when necessary. Together, they can develop a cohesive response plan that ensures all care team members are prepared to act swiftly in an emergency.

Likewise, clinical goals and QI projects often address patient satisfaction and experience. Both midwives and OB-GYNs have a role in ensuring that patients feel supported and empowered throughout their pregnancy and delivery. QI initiatives may focus on improving communication between providers and patients, enhancing shared decision-making, or increasing continuity of care across the prenatal, delivery, and postpartum stages. By collecting data through patient surveys and outcome measures, midwifery and OB-GYN teams can continually refine their practices to ensure they meet patients' needs and provide high-quality care.

## Incorporating Safety Protocols in High-Risk Management

Effective management of high-risk pregnancies is critical for ensuring maternal and fetal safety. Safety protocols are central in guiding the care provided by CNMs and OB-GYNs in cases where medical complications may arise. Incorporating well-defined safety protocols helps reduce the risk of adverse outcomes, streamline care during emergencies, and ensure that all care team members are aligned on the best course of action.

High-risk pregnancies—such as those involving preeclampsia, gestational diabetes, multiple gestations, or placental complications—require close monitoring and the ability to provide rapid care when needed. In these situations, clear and evidence-based safety protocols ensure that midwives and physicians can respond efficiently to patient condition changes.

One key aspect of incorporating safety protocols in high-risk management is the early identification of risk factors. During prenatal visits, midwives are often the first to detect signs that a pregnancy may be classified as high-risk. Having protocols that specify when to consult with or transfer care to an OB-GYN ensures that the patient receives the appropriate level of care without delay. For example, a protocol might stipulate that patients with elevated blood pressure in late pregnancy be immediately referred to a maternal-fetal medicine specialist for further evaluation. This helps prevent conditions like preeclampsia from progressing undetected.

Another crucial safety protocol component is defining each provider's roles and responsibilities during labor and delivery. For instance, if a patient develops signs of fetal distress during labor, the protocol may specify that the midwife initiates non-invasive measures to improve fetal oxygenation (e.g., repositioning the mother or providing supplemental oxygen). At the same time, the physician is notified by CNM direction to assess the need for potential surgical intervention. This clear delineation of responsibilities ensures that care is escalated appropriately and without hesitation.

Incorporating safety protocols also involves using emergency response systems, such as standardized checklists and rapid-response teams. In situations like postpartum hemorrhage, where rapid action is required to prevent maternal morbidity, having pre-established safety protocols allows the care team to act swiftly and in coordination. Midwives, physicians, and nursing staff can work together using a step-by-step approach to control bleeding, administer necessary medications, and initiate further interventions as needed. By practicing these protocols in simulation exercises (as discussed earlier), the care team can ensure they are prepared to manage these emergencies effectively.

## The Role of Feedback Loops in Improving Practice

Feedback loops are a vital component of CQI in healthcare, allowing midwives and physicians to reflect on their practices, learn from their experiences, and make informed adjustments to care delivery. By establishing a structured feedback system, hospitals can ensure that both individual providers and care teams continuously evaluate their performance and identify areas for improvement. Feedback loops involve the collection, analysis, and discussion of both positive and negative outcomes to enhance patient care and safety.

One effective way to implement feedback loops is through regular case reviews and morbidity and mortality (M and M) conferences. These forums allow midwives and OB-GYNs to review challenging or complex cases, discuss what went well, and identify areas where improvements could be made. For example, in the case of a postpartum hemorrhage that required surgical intervention, the care team might review the timeline of events to determine whether the hemorrhage was identified and managed as quickly as possible. Did the team follow established protocols? Were there any communication breakdowns that delayed care? By answering these questions, the team can refine their approach and ensure that future cases are handled more effectively.

In addition to formal case reviews, informal feedback mechanisms can be valuable in improving practice. Midwives and physicians can engage in real-time debriefings after significant events, such as an assisted delivery or a C-section. These debriefings allow the care team to reflect on their performance immediately after the event while the details remain fresh. This type of real-time feedback can help identify small but significant improvements that might not emerge in more formal reviews. For instance, the team might identify ways to improve provider handoffs or streamline communication during an emergency.

Patient feedback is another critical component of feedback loops in maternity care. Hospitals can collect patient feedback through surveys or interviews, asking mothers about their experiences with care during pregnancy, labor, and postpartum recovery. This feedback helps identify gaps in patient-centered care, such as whether the patient felt fully informed and involved in decision-making or whether her preferences were respected. Both midwives and OB-GYNs can use this feedback to improve their communication and collaboration practices, ensuring that patients have a more positive experience in the future.

Feedback loops can be strengthened through the use of data analytics. By tracking clinical outcomes such as cesarean section rates, rates of postpartum hemorrhage, or maternal satisfaction scores, hospitals can identify trends and areas for improvement. For example, suppose data shows a particular unit has higher-than-average cesarean section rates. In that case, the care team can investigate whether unnecessary interventions are being performed and develop strategies to address this issue. Data-driven feedback allows hospitals to make informed, evidence-based decisions about how to improve care quality and safety.

# Chapter 12

## Ethical Challenges in Collaborative Care and Managing Ethical Dilemmas in Patient Care

Ethical challenges are inherent in healthcare, particularly in collaborative settings where different providers bring distinct perspectives, training, and approaches to patient care. In midwifery, where patient autonomy and a low-intervention model are central, conflicts can sometimes arise between CNMs and physicians (especially OB-GYNs), who may lean more toward medical intervention. These differences can create ethical dilemmas, especially when patient preferences and clinical recommendations diverge.

One common ethical dilemma involves decision-making in high-risk pregnancies. For instance, a patient may wish to continue with a natural, low-intervention birth despite signs of emerging complications that could pose risks to her or the baby's health. Midwives, whose practice is grounded in supporting natural childbirth, may feel torn between honoring the patient's wishes and adhering to clinical guidelines that recommend intervention. In these cases, CNMs and OB-GYNs must collaborate transparently, ensuring that the patient is fully informed about the risks and benefits of her options. Informed consent is the cornerstone of ethical decision-making in healthcare, and both midwives and physicians must work together to ensure that the patient's autonomy is respected while also providing evidence-based recommendations.

Another ethical dilemma may arise in cases where the clinical judgment of the CNM and the OB-GYN differ significantly. For example, a midwife may feel that a patient can safely continue labor without intervention, while the OB-GYN may recommend a cesarean section due to concerns about fetal distress. Navigating these differing perspectives requires clear communication and a commitment to maintaining the patient's trust and ensuring her involvement in decision-making. Both providers must come to a consensus that balances the safety of the patient and the baby with the ethical obligation to respect the patient's preferences.

Midwives may also encounter ethical challenges when advocating for patients who face systemic barriers, such as lack of access to appropriate care or financial constraints. CNMs often serve as patient advocates in these cases, ensuring that vulnerable populations receive equitable care. This advocacy role sometimes puts midwives in ethical dilemmas when resources are limited or institutional policies conflict with the patient's best interests. In such scenarios, collaboration with physicians and hospital administration is crucial to finding ethical solutions prioritizing patient welfare.

# Chapter 13

# Professional Conduct and Maintaining Patient Confidentiality

In collaborative care environments, professionalism and respect between healthcare providers are essential for fostering trust and delivering quality care. One key aspect of professional conduct is the ability to work within one's scope of practice while respecting the expertise of colleagues. In a hospital setting, where CNMs and OB-GYNs often share the responsibility for patient care, professional boundaries must be clearly defined to avoid conflict. Both CNMs and physicians must recognize and value the unique contributions each brings to the care team, working together to provide a seamless, patient-centered approach to maternity care.

Maintaining patient confidentiality is another critical ethical and professional responsibility. In maternity care, where multiple providers may be involved in a patient's care, all care team members must follow strict protocols for safeguarding personal health information (PHI). This means ensuring that all communication about the patient's care is shared only with those directly involved and for legitimate clinical purposes. Any discussions about a patient's condition, preferences, or medical history should occur in private settings, such as during patient consultations or team meetings, and never in public areas.

In the digital age, maintaining confidentiality also involves safeguarding electronic health records (EHRs). Both midwives and physicians must adhere to HIPAA regulations, ensuring that patient information is accessed only when necessary and that proper encryption and security measures are in place. Whether intentional or accidental, breaches of patient confidentiality can undermine the trust between the patient and her providers and lead to legal consequences for the hospital and the individual healthcare provider.

In collaborative care models, it's also essential that healthcare providers maintain clear and respectful communication with patients and colleagues. When discussing sensitive medical information or addressing differing opinions, professionalism dictates that all interactions remain respectful, evidence-based, and focused on the patient's best interests. Disparaging remarks or undermining a colleague in front of a patient damages the professional relationship and erodes the patient's confidence in her care team.

Hence, professional conduct and ethical decision-making in collaborative care settings ensure that both the patient's safety and her autonomy are protected. By fostering mutual respect and maintaining confidentiality, CNMs and OB-GYNs can work together to provide the best possible care.

## Collaboration in Birth Work within Hospitals

Collaboration between CNMs and OB-GYNs is essential in hospital settings to ensure comprehensive, patient-centered care. This teamwork enhances routine and high-risk maternity care, combining the midwives' focus on natural and low-intervention childbirth with the physicians' expertise in managing complications and performing surgical interventions.

Training and education are key to effective collaboration. Orientation programs for OB residents introduce them to midwifery practices. In contrast, joint simulation exercises and mentorship programs help midwives and physicians develop a shared understanding of their roles and responsibilities. Regular case reviews and morbidity and mortality conferences strengthen this collaborative approach, allowing the care team to reflect on their performance and improve clinical outcomes.

In high-risk pregnancies, clear communication and safety protocols guide the collaborative efforts of CNMs and OB-GYNs, ensuring timely and appropriate care. Structured communication tools like SBAR (Situation, Background, Assessment, Recommendation) help streamline information exchange and decision-making processes.

Maintaining continuous patient engagement is also crucial. Midwives often serve as the primary point of contact, providing emotional and physical support throughout the patient's journey. This continuity of care, combined with shared decision-making, ensures that patients' preferences and autonomy are respected, even in complex medical situations.

By fostering mutual respect, adhering to professional conduct, and prioritizing patient confidentiality, midwives and physicians can work together effectively to deliver high-quality maternity care. This collaborative model enhances patient safety and satisfaction and creates a supportive and efficient healthcare environment.

# References


- American College of Nurse-Midwives (ACNM). (2012). Standards for the Practice of Midwifery. ACNM. https://www.midwife.org/Standards
- American College of Nurse-Midwives (ACNM). (2021). Midwifery Workforce and Education. ACNM. https://www.midwife.org/Midwifery-Workforce-and-Education
- American College of Obstetricians and Gynecologists (ACOG). (2016). Collaboration in Practice: Implementing Team-Based Care. ACOG Committee Opinion No. 657. https://www.acog.org/clinical/clinical-guidance/committee-opinion/articles/2016/02/collaboration-in-practice-implementing-team-based-care
- American College of Obstetricians and Gynecologists (ACOG). (2019). Levels of Maternal Care. ACOG Obstetric Care Consensus No. 9. https://www.acog.org/clinical/clinical-guidance/obstetric-care-consensus/articles/2019/02/levels-of-maternal-care
- Bohren, M. A., Hofmeyr, G. J., Sakala, C., Fukuzawa, R. K., and Cuthbert, A. (2017). Continuous support for women during childbirth. Cochrane Database of Systematic Reviews, 7. https://doi.org/10.1002/14651858.CD003766.pub6
- Homer, C. S., Friberg, I. K., Dias, M. A., et al. (2014). The projected effect of scaling up midwifery. The Lancet, 384(9948), 1146-1157. https://doi.org/10.1016/S0140-6736(14)60790-X
- Institute for Healthcare Improvement (IHI). (2019). The Continuous Quality Improvement (CQI) Process. IHI.

http://www.ihi.org/resources/Pages/HowtoImprove/ScienceofImprovementHowtoImprove.aspx

- Kirkpatrick, H., Cantrell, M., and Smeltzer, S. C. (2018). Interprofessional Collaboration and Education in Maternity Care. Journal of Obstetric, Gynecologic and Neonatal Nursing, 47(5), 652-659. https://doi.org/10.1016/j.jogn.2018.06.006
- McDonald, S., Grant, A., Sheridan, E., et al. (2016). Midwifery-led continuity models and collaborative maternity care. Journal of Midwifery and Women's Health, 61(6), 688-698. https://doi.org/10.1111/jmwh.12495
- Reiner, G., and MacDonald, J. (2015). Collaborative Practice in Maternity Care: Cross-Disciplinary Approaches to Care. Journal of Perinatal and Neonatal Nursing, 29(1), 68-75. https://doi.org/10.1097/JPN.0000000000000068
- Sandall, J., Soltani, H., Gates, S., Shennan, A., and Devane, D. (2016). Midwife-led continuity models versus other models of care for childbearing women. Cochrane Database of Systematic Reviews, 4.https://doi.org/10.1002/14651858.CD004667.pub5
- The Joint Commission. (2020). Sentinel Event Alert: Preventing maternal deaths. The Joint Commission. https://www.jointcommission.org/
- The National Institute for Health and Care Excellence (NICE). (2014). Intrapartum care: care of healthy women and their babies during childbirth. NICE Clinical Guideline. https://www.nice.org.uk/guidance/cg190
- The Royal College of Midwives. (2016). Better Births: Improving outcomes of maternity services in England. National Maternity Review.

https://www.england.nhs.uk/publication/better-births-improving-outcomes-of-maternity-services-in-england/

World Health Organization (WHO). (2016). WHO Recommendations: Intrapartum care for a positive childbirth experience. WHO. https://www.who.int/publications-detail/9789241550215

# MD/CNM Communication: Consultation, Collaboration & Referral Guide

This document outlines communication protocols and patient care responsibilities between CNMs and MDs across labor, delivery, and postpartum scenarios. The aim is clear, effective, and collaborative clinical decision-making.

---

**Level I – Shift Report**

Purpose: To ensure transparency between teams and proactively address patient care needs and anticipated issues.

**Discuss:**

- **Labors:** Inductions, augmentations, present all medical conditions affecting the pregnancy
- **Postpartum:** Anticipated discharges
- **Admissions:** Anticipated, with bed availability
- **Potential Issues:**
    - Macrosomia (plan for MD involvement at transition or 2nd stage)
    - Potential Cesarean (MD availability or CNM first-assist)

Both CNM and MD teams report during shift change.

---

**Level II – Consultation**

**Definition:** CNM seeks guidance from MD; CNM retains primary care responsibility. MD documents consult and any plan changes. Disagreements escalated to service directors.

**Scenarios:**

- **Inductions:**
    - <41 weeks post-dates with ood dating
    - Social inductions (CNM-to-CNM first, then MD)
- **Fetal Demise (2nd/3rd trimester):** CNM patients only; discuss labs, complications, delivery support
- **Inadequate Labor Progress:**
    - 1st Stage: No change after 4 hrs of adequate contractions
    - 2nd Stage:
        - Primip: >4 hrs (or >6 hrs w/ epidural)
        - Multip: >4 hr (or >6 hrs w/ epidural)
    - 3rd Stage: >30 mins or excessive bleeding
- **Other Triggers:**
    - Non-reassuring FHT patterns unresponsive to intervention
    - Maternal temp >100.4°F
    - U/S abnormalities (fibroids, size/date issues, IUGR, AFI abnormalities)
    - 3rd trimester bleeding (no previa or cervicitis)
    - History of 2 preterm births or <2500g infants
    - Hepatitis C (after MD eval, if no active liver disease)
    - Intrahepatic cholestasis of pregnancy

---

**Level III – Collaboration**

**Definition:** CNM and MD jointly manage care. MD may assume primary responsibility during critical periods, with CNM continuing in a supportive/clinical role.

**Scenarios:**

- Arrest of labor unresponsive to CNM measures

- Abnormal presentation/lie >37 weeks
    - May return to CNM care if ECV successful
- Severe PPH or retained placenta
- Extensive lacerations (3rd/4th degree) – depends on CNM skill
- Mild preeclampsia
- Stillbirth
- No prenatal care at labor admission
    - May remain under CNM after MD assessment
- Antepartum severe anemia
- Postpartum BTL
    - CNM manages remainder of IP care
- Vaginal delivery from Level II labor
    - CNM may resume postpartum care and laceration repair

---

**Level IV – Transfer of Care**

**Definition:** MD or perinatologist assumes full care responsibility. Must be documented.

**Scenarios:**

- Serious fetal anomalies
- Chronic hypertension (requiring medication)
- Multiple gestation
- IDDM or A2 GDM
- Severe medical comorbidities:
    - Lupus/collagen vascular disease
    - Seizure disorders
    - Heart disease / arrhythmias (unless cleared by cardiologist)

- HIV/AIDS
- Uncontrolled thyroid, liver, renal disease
- Active TB
- Hepatitis C with abnormal LFTs
- Moderate-severe asthma

- Isoimmunization
- Preterm labor with cervical change not halted by hydration/meds
- Severe preeclampsia/eclampsia
- Prolapsed cord
- Cesarean delivery
    - CNM may round or perform 8-week PP visit
- Family planning education remains CNM role (with MD note)
- **Antepartum Transfers:**
    - Persistent previa >28 weeks
    - Planned repeat CD (mid-3rd trimester)
    - Two prior CDs (considered VBAC)
    - Active HSV at labor
    - BMI >45 or projected >45 at delivery

---

**Conditions Requiring Early MD Involvement or Transfer**

**Immediate Transfer to MD Service:**

- 2 uterine scars with no prior vaginal delivery
- Classical cesarean or myomectomy
- Placenta previa at 32 weeks
- Pre-pregnancy BMI ≥50
- A1c >8% in early 2nd trimester for diabetics

- Mono-mono twins
- Any uncontrolled or high-risk maternal conditions requiring advanced care

**Antepartum Physician Consult Required:**

- Pregestational diabetes (by 20w)
- Non-vertex/vertex twins (by 36w)
- Malpresentation at term (by 36w)
- History of low transverse C-section (28–32w)

---

**Management of Specific Conditions**

**Prior Low Transverse Cesarean (TOLAC Candidates):**

- **28–32w:** MD consult, TOLAC consent prior to visit
- **38w:** Optional MD consult to assess pelvis
- **Admission Requirements:**
  - Saline lock IV
  - Continuous EFM
  - Resident coverage

**Malpresentation @ 36 Weeks:**

- MD consult for ECV vs. scheduled CD
- ECV scheduled post-37w at BUMCP
- If scheduled for CD, patient should see operating MD beforehand

**Twins:**

- Non-vertex/vertex twins require MD consult at 36w
- Physician presence strongly preferred for all twin vaginal deliveries
  - Physician is required to be present for delivery

---

**Admission & Intrapartum Communication**

**Preterm Admission (<37w):**

- **<34w:** Must transfer to MD care
- **34–37w:** CNM consults MD; CNM may retain care

**Term Labor Admission:**

- Notify MD via text:
    - G/P, EGA, SVE, Room
    - Comorbidities
- Send H&P if consultation initiated
- **CNM Admission Note Must Include:**
    - Collaborating physician role
    - Documentation of MD notification and plan

**Notify MD by Phone if:**

- Severe-range BPs or magnesium started
- Persistent Cat II FHTs
- Second stage exceeds 3 hours
- Instrumental or cesarean delivery likely
- 3rd/4th degree lacerations
- Stage II PPH or requiring assistance
- Any complications or concerns

---

**Postpartum Rounds & Disposition**

- CNMs will see their own patients unless otherwise arranged.
- Text physician post-rounds with patient status (room #, discharge plan).
- Call MD for any complications or concerns.

---

**Definitions**

**Transfer of Care:** Physician takes full responsibility. CNM documents transfer; MD assumes clinical decisions and orders. CNM may continue in support role.
**Consultation:** Physician input requested; MD may or may not see patient. Documentation must reflect the discussion and any recommendations.
**Sample Physician Addendum:** *"I have discussed the care of this patient with CNM and agree with plan. Recommendations: [X]. I am in-house and immediately available if needed."*

# Focused Clinical Guide

**The following conditions require <u>consultation</u> with the collaborating physician:**

a. Gestation age greater than 42 weeks
b. Preeclampsia
c. Substance abuse (current)
d. Intrauterine fetal demise in current or previous pregnancy
e. History of intrauterine growth restriction in previous pregnancy (<5%tile). If normal growth is documented by serial ultrasound mensuration in current pregnancy, consultation may not be required.
f. Uterine anomalies
g. Symptomatic anemia or hematocrit ≤21% / hemoglobin ≤7g
h. Evidence of syphilis at any stage
i. Oligohydramnios or polyhydramnios, documented by ultrasound
j. Evidence of fetal abnormality. The collaborating physician may change to transfer status based on the nature of the abnormality.
k. Intrauterine growth restriction in current pregnancy.
l. A2DM in good control
m. History of shoulder dystocia
n. Premature labor – less than 37 weeks.
o. Suspected fetal macrosomia, defined as an estimated fetal weight over 4500g in diabetics or over 5000g in non-diabetics.
p. BMI > 40
q. History of bariatric (weight loss) surgery
r. Previous unexplained neonatal mortality or stillbirth
s. Absent prenatal care at term
t. History of seizure disorder in adulthood
u. History of HELLP
v. History of uterine surgery, including myomectomy
w. One prior cesarean birth with low transverse incision
x. Significant history of or current cardiovascular, renal, hepatic, neurological or severe gastrointestinal disorder or disease
y. Significant history of or current endocrine disorder (excluding controlled mild hypothyroidism)
z. Pulmonary disease/active tuberculosis/severe asthma
aa. Collagen vascular diseases
bb. Significant hematological disorders
cc. Current or recent diagnosis of cancer requiring chemotherapy
dd. History of cervical cerclage
ee. Trial of Labor After Cesarean (TOLAC):
    1) For all TOLAC patients the Collaborating Physician is

required to remain on campus during the active phase of labor (5-6 cm).

2) The CNM may document progress notes in the medical record, as well as the Admission, History and Physical and Informed Consent for a TOLAC patient.
3) The CNM may perform routine exams, AROM, and placement of internal monitors of a patient undergoing a TOLAC, in collaboration with the physician.
4) The CNM may perform the delivery of the patient undergoing a TOLAC, at the discretion of the physician, who shall be present on the unit and immediately available for assistance. Delivery notes completed by the CNM.

ff. During labor:
1) Persistent Category II heart rate changes
2) Arrest of active phase in which change in cervical dilation has not been demonstrated after 4 hours of an adequate uterine contraction plan.
3) Prolonged 2nd stage of labor. A prolonged second stage of labor warrants clinical reassessment of the patient, fetus, and expulsive forces. As per ACOG Guidelines.
4) Prolonged rupture of membranes > 18 hours.
5) Elevated temperature (>38 degrees C) or evidence of chorioamnionitis

gg. During Delivery:
1) Significant lacerations
2) Need for manual removal of placenta, or if placenta is retained after 30 minutes.
3) Post-partum or intrapartum hemorrhage

This is not an all-inclusive list and other conditions may arise that require consultation, including a change in maternal or fetal status.

**The following conditions require <u>transfer</u> to the collaborating physician:**

**Transfer will consist of the transfer of the care of the pregnant patient to the collaborating physician, who will be directly responsible for the management of the condition(s). The CNM may continue to provide nursing care, labor and delivery support and delivery to the patient and may assist in subsequent c-section as first or second-assist, depending on OR experience and training.**

a. Previous uterine surgery which requires a cesarean delivery.
b. Malpresentation at term.
c. Placenta previa.
d. Abruptio placentae or significant bleeding.

e. Diabetes mellitus, other than well controlled Class A2DM
f. Multiple gestation.
g. Category III fetal heart rate tracings.
h. Current Preeclampsia with severe features, eclampsia, HELLP syndrome and related conditions.
i. Evidence of "TORCH" primary infection.
j. Vulvar, vaginal or cervical lesions suspicious of herpes genitalia.
k. Failed home delivery and "no doc' obstetrical patients. The collaborating physician may reassign these patients to "consultation" status following in-house physical assessment of the patient.
l. Any condition requiring a cesarean section or surgical intervention.
m. Severe or uncontrolled maternal medical conditions which require a higher level of decision making or management.

www.ingramcontent.com/pod-product-compliance
Lightning Source LLC
LaVergne TN
LVHW022306200926
848481LV00004B/1230
* 9 7 9 8 8 6 9 3 4 8 1 2 8 *